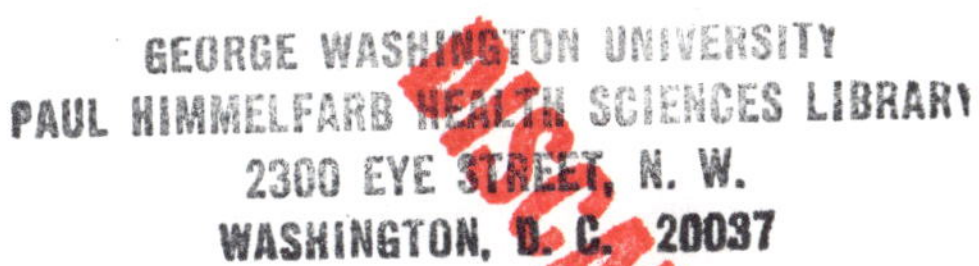

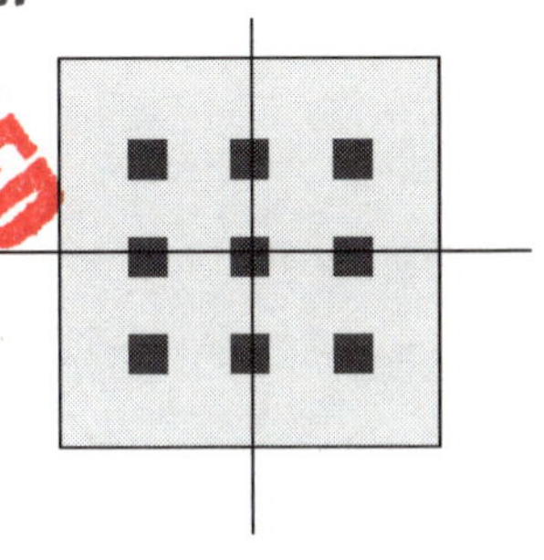

Laboratory Testing in Ob/Gyn

EDITED BY

Gerald D. Willett, MD

*Assistant Professor, Department of Obstetrics and Gynecology
and Pathology*
Georgetown University Medical Center
Washington, DC

BOSTON

Blackwell Scientific Publications

OXFORD • LONDON • EDINBURGH
MELBOURNE • PARIS • BERLIN • VIENNA

Blackwell Scientific Publications

EDITORIAL OFFICES:
238 Main Street, Cambridge, Massachusetts
  02142, USA
Osney Mead, Oxford OX2 0EL, England
25 John Street, London WC1N 2BL, England
23 Ainslie Place, Edinburgh EH3 6AJ,
  Scotland
54 University Street, Carlton, Victoria 3053,
  Australia
Arnette SA, 1 rue de Lille, 75007 Paris,
  France
Blackwell-Wissenschaft, Düsseldorfer Str. 38,
  D-10707, Berlin, Germany
Blackwell MZV, Feldgasse 13, A-1238
  Vienna, Austria

DISTRIBUTORS:
USA
Blackwell Scientific Publications
238 Main Street
Cambridge, Massachusetts 02142
(Telephone orders: 800-215-1000 or 617-
  876-7000)

Canada
Times Mirror Professional Publishing
130 Flaska Drive
Markham, Ontario L6G 1B8
(Telephone orders: 800-268-4178 or 905-
  470-6739)

Australia
Blackwell Scientific Publications (Australia)
  Pty Ltd
54 University Street
Carlton, Victoria 3053
(Telephone orders: 03-347-5552)

Outside North America and Australia
Blackwell Scientific Publications, Ltd.
c/o Marston Book Services, Ltd.
P.O. Box 87
Oxford OX2 0DT, England
(Telephone orders: 44-865-791155)

Typeset by Huron Valley Graphics
Printed and bound by Braun-Brumfield, Inc.

*Library of Congress Cataloging-in-
Publication Data*

Laboratory testing in ob/gyn / edited by
Gerald D. Willett.
    p.   cm.
    Includes bibliographical references and
    index.
    ISBN 0-86542-290-7 :
    1. Obstetrics—Diagnosis.
    2. Gynecology—Diagnosis.
    3. Laboratory diagnosis. I. Willett,
    Gerald D.
    [DNLM: 1. Genital Diseases,
Female—diagnosis. 2. Pregnancy
    Complications—diagnosis.
3. Obstetrics. 4. Gynecology.
  5. Chemistry, Clinical—methods.
WP 141 L1235 1994]
    RG527.5.L3L33   1994
    618'.0475—dc20
    DNLM/DLC
    for Library of Congress   94-7677
                                          CIP
                                          r94

Contents

iii

Contributors

Robert L. Barbieri, MD: Kate Macy Ladd Professor of Obstetrics, Gynecology, and Reproductive Biology, Harvard Medical School; Chairman of Obstetrics and Gynecology, Brigham and Women's Hospital, Boston, Massachusetts

Willard A. Barnes, MD: Associate Professor and Director, Division of Gynecologic Oncology, Department of Obstetrics and Gynecology, Vincent T. Lombardi Cancer Research Center, Georgetown University Medical Center, Washington, DC

James F. Barter, MD: Associate Professor, Division of Gynecologic Oncology, Department of Obstetrics and Gynecology, Vincent T. Lombardi, Cancer Research Center, Georgetown University Medical Center, Washington, DC

Sarah L. Berga, MD: Assistant Professor, Division of Reproductive Endocrinology, Departments of Obstetrics, Gynecology and Reproductive Sciences and of Psychiatry, University of Pittsburgh School of Medicine, Pittsburgh, Pennsylvania

Karin J. Blakemore, MD: Associate Professor, Division of Maternal-Fetal Medicine, Department of Gynecology and Obstetrics, The Johns Hopkins University School of Medicine, Baltimore, Maryland

Berry A. Campbell, MD: Assistant Professor, Maternal-Fetal Medicine, University of Kentucky Medical Center, Lexington, Kentucky

Larry J. Copeland, MD: Professor of Obstetrics and Gynecology, Director, Gynecologic Oncology, The Ohio State University College of Medicine, Columbus, Ohio

Susan M. Cox, MD: Associate Professor, Department of Obstetrics and Gynecology, University of Texas Southwestern Medical Center, Dallas, Texas

Bonnie J. Dattel, MD: Director, Research and Education, Associate Professor, Maternal-Fetal Medicine, Eastern Virginia Medical School, Medical College of Hampton Roads, Norfolk, Virginia

Edward C. Grendys, Jr., MD: Instructor, Division of Gynecologic Oncology, Department of Obstetrics and Gynecology, Georgetown University Medical Center, Washington, DC

Nicolette S. Horbach, MD: Assistant Professor and Director, Division of Gynecology and Uro-Gynecology, George Washington University Medical Center, Washington, DC

J. A. James, MD: Medical Director, Perinatal Center of Wisconsin, Milwaukee, Wisconsin

George T. Koulianos, MD: Clinical Assistant Professor, Department of Obstetrics and Gynecology, University of South Alabama, Mobile, Alabama

Shaun G. Lencki, MD: Instructor, Division of Maternal-Fetal Medicine, Department of Obstetrics and Gynecology, Georgetown University School of Medicine, Washington, DC

George S. Lewandowski, MD: Assistant Professor, Department of Obstetrics and Gynecology, Division of Gynecologic Oncology, Arthur G. James Cancer Hospital and Research Institute, The Ohio State University College of Medicine, Columbus, Ohio

Everett F. Magann, MD: Division of Maternal-Fetal Medicine, Department of Obstetrics and Gynecology, University of Mississippi Medical Center, Jackson, Mississippi

Sanford M. Markham, MD: Assistant Professor, Division of Reproductive Endocrinology and Infertility, Department of Obstetrics and Gynecology, Georgetown University Medical Center, Washington, DC

James N. Martin, Jr., MD: Professor and Director, Division of Maternal-Fetal Medicine, Department of Obstetrics and Gynecology, University of Mississippi Medical Center, Jackson, Mississippi

Kathryn D. McGowan, MD: Assistant Professor of Obstetrics and Gynecology, Division of Biology and Medicine, Brown University; Director, Prenatal Diagnostic Center of Women and Infants Hospital of Rhode Island, Providence, Rhode Island

Susan Marie Mou, MD: Associate Professor, Department of Obstetrics and Gynecology, University of Missouri School of Medicine, Truman Medical Center, Kansas City, Missouri

P. J. Osypowski, MT: Department of Obstetrics and Gynecology, Sinai Samaritan Medical Center, Milwaukee, Wisconsin

Thomas L. Pinckert, MD: Assistant Professor, Co-Chief, Division of Genetics, Division of Maternal-Fetal Medicine, Department of Obstetrics and Gynecology, Georgetown University School of Medicine, Washington, DC

Ronald K. Potkul, MD: Associate Professor, Director, Division of Gynecologic Oncology, Department of Obstetrics and Gynecology, Loyola University Medical Center, Chicago, Illinois

John T. Queenan, MD: Professor and Chairman, Department of Obstetrics and Gynecology, Georgetown University Medical Center, Washington, DC

Periclis Roussis, MD: Director, Fort Sanders Perinatal Center, Knoxville, Tennessee

Preston C. Sacks, MD: Division of Fertility and Reproductive Endocrinology, Columbia Hospital for Women; Clinical Instructor, Department of Obstetrics and Gynecology, Georgetown University School of Medicine, Washington, DC

Nancy J. Scaglione, MD: WomenNow Health Care, S.C., Milwaukee, Wisconsin

Anthony R. Scialli, MD: Department of Obstetrics and Gynecology, Georgetown University Medical Center, Washington, DC

James A. Simon, MD: Associate Professor and Chief, Division of Reproductive Endocrinology and Infertility, Department of Obstetrics and Gynecology, Georgetown University Medical Center, Washington, DC

Jessica L. Thomason, MD: Professor of Obstetrics and Gynecology, University of Wisconsin School of Medicine; Medical Director, WomenNow Health Care, S.C., Milwaukee, Wisconsin

Ian H. Thorneycroft, MD, PhD: Professor and Chairman, Department of Obstetrics and Gynecology, University of South Alabama, Mobile, Alabama

James P. Toner, MD, PhD: Jones Institute for Reproductive Medicine, Department of Obstetrics and Gynecology, Eastern Virginia Medical School, Norfolk, Virginia

Kathy A. Trumbull, MD: Instructor, Division of Reproductive Endocrinology and Infertility, Department of Obstetrics and Gynecology, Georgetown University Medical Center, Washington, DC

Gail F. Whitman, MD: Assistant Professor, Section of Reproductive Endocrinology, Infertility, and Genetics, Department of Obstetrics and Gynecology, Medical College of Georgia, Augusta, Georgia

Barry I. Witten, MD: Director, Reproductive Endocrinology, Assistant Clinical Professor, Department of Obstetrics and Gynecology, St. Johns Mercy Medical Center, St. Louis, Missouri

Gerald D. Willett, MD: Assistant Professor, Departments of Obstetrics and Gynecology and Pathology, Georgetown University Medical Center, Washington, DC

Michael J. Zinaman, MD: Associate Professor, Director, Division of Reproductive Endocrinology and Infertility, Department of Obstetrics and Gynecology, Loyola University Medical Center, Chicago, Illinois

Preface

Many excellent texts have been written discussing anatomic pathology in obstetrics and gynecology. This book, in distinction, focuses on the role of the clinical laboratory in our specialty.

The chapters have been selected to emphasize commonly performed tests, clinical problems requiring multiple or sequential testing, basic laboratory principles, and lab alterations secondary to medications.

The test section in the second half of the book lists the laboratory tests in alphabetical order. Information regarding specimen collection, reference range, and clinical correlations are provided. This section is meant to complement and not duplicate the information provided in the initial chapters.

It is important that the clinician consult his own laboratory for the reference range at his institution. Many of these tests have multiple methodologies. Newer methods are constantly being introduced. Though emphasis on incorporating international units appears to be waning in some of the U.S. journals, these units are provided in parentheses. In addition to lab tests, the test section also includes a listing of infectious organisms along with the tests that lead to their identification.

I would like to express my sincere appreciation to the contributing authors and especially to Dr. John Queenan who provided continuous support in preparing this work. Many thanks also are extended to previous mentors and colleagues—Dr. Frederick Kraus, Dr. James Blythe, Dr. John Anstey, Dr. William Hughes, and Dr. Robert Kurman. My greatest debt is to my wife Terri, who relinquished the home computer and many hours to allow for completion of this work.

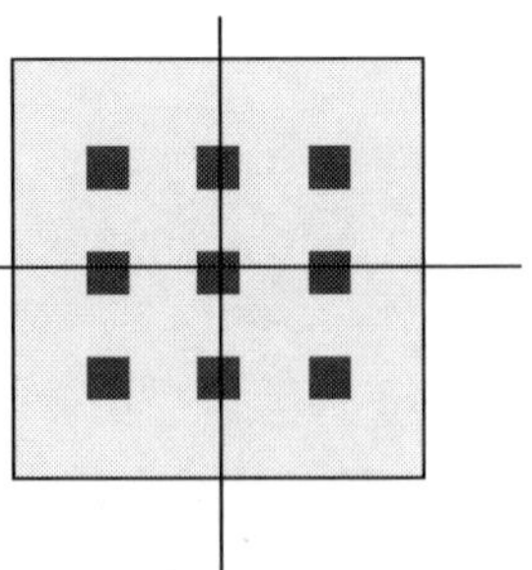

PART ONE

General Health Care and Routine Prenatal Laboratory Determinations

1.
Health Maintenance

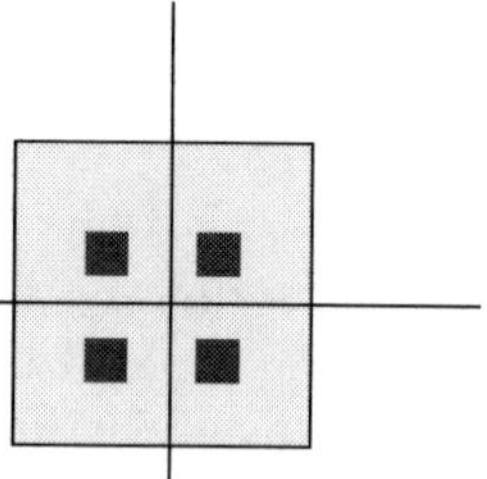

Gerald D. Willett

The most common laboratory testing performed by obstetrician-gynecologists for health maintenance includes Pap smears, cholesterol screening, fecal occult blood screening, and prenatal testing.

Pap Smear

The Pap smear is among the most common laboratory tests performed for preventive health care in women. It is also one of the most effective screening tests in medical care. Significant decreases in the frequency of cervical cancer have occurred since the inception of mass screening in the 1940s. Although earlier cost-effectiveness studies encouraged more extended time intervals between Pap smears (after three normal annual evaluations), most obstetrician-gynecologists recommend yearly screening for their patients. Initial evaluation should begin at age 18 (1) or when a woman becomes sexually active. Annual screening for women also allows for evaluation of many other aspects of health care in addition to gynecologic problems.

Proper collection techniques include adequate sampling of both the cervical transformation zone and the endocervical canal. A combination of the Ayre spatula and a brush instrument will provide a satisfactory smear in most cases. Discharge and small amounts of blood should be gently removed from the cervix before sampling. Sampling the ectocervix first may help to avoid the bleeding that the brush occasionally elicits. Endocervical preparations may be improved by first removing thick tenacious mucus with an additional brush. Rapid fixation should be used to prevent air-drying artifact. Wet smear preparation, gonococcal, and chlamydial testing should be performed liberally to evaluate abnormal discharge.

At the end of 1988, a group of cytologic and clinical experts formulated a consensus classification for cervicovaginal cytology in the United States. Cytology laboratories had been using different modifications of Papanicolaou's numbered classification. The principal refinements of the new classification, termed the Bethesda system (2,3), used descriptive terminology, placed special emphasis on specimen adequacy, and made modifications in the classification of squamous abnormalities. Table 1-1 presents the basic structure of the Bethesda classification. Additional clinical correlations can be found in Part 7.

Cholesterol Screening

Coronary heart disease (CHD) is a major health problem for women, accounting for approximately 25% of all deaths. The risk of CHD approximately doubles after menopause. Cholesterol screening measurements are important determinations of risk for CHD. The first steps in patient evaluation are risk assessment for CHD and measurement of nonfasting total cholesterol. Risk factors include hypertension, diabetes mellitus, cigarette smoking, severe obesity, cerebrovascular and peripheral vascular disease, and family history of premature CHD.

For the patient whose total cholesterol level is $\geq$ 200 mg/dL rescreening should be performed in 5 years (4). A confirmed total cholesterol level of 200–239 mg/dL is considered borderline. If no risk factors are present, dietary information should be provided and the total cholesterol determination should be repeated in one year. If risk factors are present, the patient should have a fasting lipoprotein evaluation.

A confirmed total cholesterol level of $\geq$ 240 mg/dL is considered to be high risk. A 12-hour fasting lipoprotein evaluation should be ordered. The laboratory determinations performed in a lipoprotein analysis include total cholesterol, high-density lipoprotein (HDL) cholesterol, low-density lipoprotein (LDL) cholesterol, and triglycerides.

Low-density lipoprotein cholesterol determinations are used as the next step in guiding management. Levels $<$ 130 mg/dL are desirable, levels of 130–159 mg/dL are borderline, and levels of $\geq$ 160 mg/dL are high risk. If the patient has no significant risk factors, the minimal goal is to obtain levels $<$ 160 mg/dL. With risk factors, the goal is to obtain LDL cholesterol levels $<$ 130 mg/dL. Dietary regimens restricting saturated fat and

TABLE 1-1. Bethesda classification

A. Description of specimen adequacy

1. Satisfactory for evaluation
2. Satisfactory but limited by. . . .*
3. Unsatisfactory for evaluation due to. . . .*
    (*blood, inflammation, artifact, cytolysis, scant specimen)

B. General categories

1. Within normal limits
2. Benign cellular changes
    a. Infection includes *Trichomonas vaginalis,* fungal organisms, coccobacilli predominance (shift in bacterial flora), *Actinomyces* species, herpes, other
    b. Reactive changes associated with inflammation, atrophy, radiation, intrauterine device, other
3. Epithelial abnormalities
    a. Squamous cell abnormality
        -Atypia of undetermined significance
           (qualify. . . . favoring reactive vs neoplastic)
        -Low-grade squamous intraepithelial lesion
        -High-grade squamous intraepithelial lesion
        -Squamous cell carcinoma
    b. Glandular cell abnormality
        -Endometrial cells in postmenopausal woman
        -Atypia of undetermined significance
        -Endocervical adenocarcinoma
        -Endometrial adenocarcinoma
        -Extrauterine carcinoma
4. Other malignant neoplasms (ie, sarcoma, lymphoma)

C. Hormonal evaluation

1. Compatible with age and history
2. Incompatible with age and history
3. Evaluation not possible due to. . . .

cholesterol are usually attempted first. Medications are used if the dietary changes do not bring the cholesterol levels down to appropriate levels (usually within 6 months).

One of the criticisms of the initial screening for total cholesterol is that it may miss some individuals with a low HDL ($<$ 35 mg/dL; 5). Low HDL is a separate risk factor for CHD.

Fecal Occult Blood Screening

The testing of stool specimens for blood dates back to 1864 when Van Deen used gum guaiac as an indicator. The American Cancer Society screening recommendations advise fecal occult blood testing annually and sigmoidoscopy every 3–5 years starting at age 50 (6). Despite low sensitivities reported for fecal occult blood screening (7), a recent study found that the screening did reduce mortality from colorectal cancer (8).

Fecal occult blood testing usually determines the peroxidase activity

---

TABLE 1-2. Prenatal testing

First Trimester	*Second Trimester*	*Third Trimester*
Pap smear	MSAFP (14–16 wk)	
Blood type	Glucose screen (24–28 wk)	
Rh	Amniocentesis	
Urinalysis	Urine protein*	Urine protein*
Urine culture	(each visit)	(each visit)
CBC	Hgb/Hct	Hgb/Hct
Antibody screen		Repeat STD
Syphilis testing		evaluation for
Rubella titer		risk groups
Gonococcal/chlamydial		
infection		
HIV (informed consent)		
Chorionic villous sampling		
Hepatitis screen		
Tuberculosis skin test		

*Some clinicians may just follow weight gain and blood pressure determinations
CBC, complete blood count; Hgb/Hct, hemoglobin/hematocrit; HIV, human immunodeficiency virus; MSAFP, maternal serum α-fetoprotein; STD, sexually transmitted disease

from red blood cells. Other methods use either immunologic techniques or a conversion of hemoglobin to fluorescent porphyrin (HemoQuant®—SmithKline Diagnostics, Philadelphia). Normally an individual loses about 2.0 mL of blood daily into the gastrointestinal tract. Testing is designed to pick up larger amounts of blood. The most widely used test is Hemoccult II® (SmithKline Diagnostics, Philadelphia), which has a relatively low amount of false positive results.

It is recommended that the patient abstain from meat, irritative medication, certain foods with high peroxidase activity, and vitamin C for 3 days prior to testing. The patient should take two samples from each of three consecutive stool specimens and submit them without excess delay for testing. A single positive determination from the fecal occult testing requires additional testing with radiologic and direct imaging procedures.

Prenatal Laboratory Testing

Table 1-2 lists commonly performed prenatal tests. Additional clinical correlations for the individual tests are presented in Part 7.

References

1. American College of Obstetricians and Gynecologists. Cervical cytology: evaluation and management of abnormalities. Technical Bulletin no. 81, 1984.
2. National Cancer Institute Workshop. The 1988 Bethesda system for reporting cervical/vaginal cytologic diagnoses. JAMA 1989;262:931–934.
3. Rapid Communication. The Bethesda system for reporting cervical/vaginal cytologic diagnoses—Report of the 1991 Bethesda Workshop. JAMA 1992; 267:1892.
4. The National Cholesterol Education Program, National Heart, Lung, and Blood Institute. Report of the National Cholesterol Education Program expert panel on detection, evaluation, and treatment of high blood cholesterol in adults. Arch Intern Med 1988;148:36–69.
5. Bush TL, Riedel D. Screening for total cholesterol. Do the National Cholesterol Education Program's recommendations detect individuals at high risk of coronary heart disease? Circulation 1991;83:1287–1293.
6. Mettlin C, Dodd GD. The American Cancer Society guidelines for the cancer-related checkup: an update. CA 1991;41:279–282.
7. Alquist, DA, Wienad HS, Moertel CG, et al. Accuracy of fecal occult blood screening for colorectal neoplasia. JAMA 1993;269:1262–1267.
8. Mandel JS, Bond JH, Church TR, et al. Reducing mortality from colorectal cancer by screening for fecal occult blood. N Engl J Med 1993;328:1365–1371.

Suggested Reading

Alquist DA, McGill DB, Schwartz S, et al. Fecal blood levels in health and disease: a study using HemoQuant. N Engl J Med 1985;312:1422–1428.

Bush TL, Barrett-Connor E, Cown LD, et al. Cardiovascular mortality and noncontraceptive use of estrogen in women: results from the Lipid Research Clinics' program follow-up study. Circulation 1987;75:1102–1109.

Frommer DJ, Kapparis A, Brown MK. Improved screening for colorectal cancer by immunological detection of occult blood. Br Med J [Clin Res] 1988;296:1092–1094.

Gnauck R, Macrae FA, Fleisher M. How to perform the fecal occult blood test. CA 1984;34:134.

Goff BA, Atanasoff P, Brown E, Muntz HG, Bell DA, Rice LW. Endocervical glandular atypia in Papanicolaou smears. Obstet Gynecol 1992;79:101–104.

Kannel WB. Metabolic risk factors for coronary heart disease in women: perspective from the Framingham study. Am Heart J 1987;114:413–419.

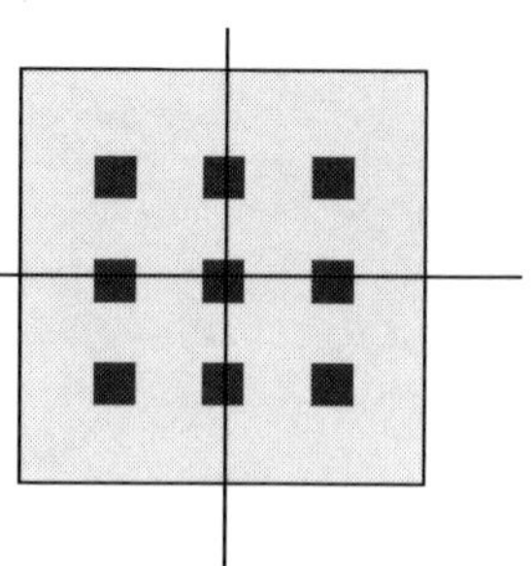

PART TWO
Obstetrics

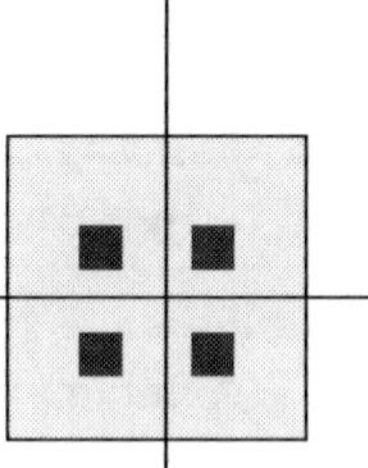

2.

Hypertensive Gravidas

Everett F. Magann
James N. Martin, Jr.

Hypertension affects 7% to 10% of all pregnancies and complicates as many as 20% to 40% of pregnancies that have underlying vascular or renal disease (1,2). Hypertensive disorders of pregnancy are further subclassified into chronic hypertension, preeclampsia/eclampsia (includes HELLP syndrome of hemolysis, elevated liver enzymes, and low platelets), preeclampsia superimposed on chronic hypertension, and gestational hypertension.

Chronic hypertension is diagnosed when hypertension exists in the nonpregnant state or is present before midgestation. Preeclampsia is defined as the triad of proteinuria ($> 1+$), nondependent edema, and pregnancy-induced hypertension ($\geq$ 140/90 mm Hg in a woman previously normotensive) occurring in the second half of pregnancy or puerperium. A preeclamptic patient with seizures unrelated to any other etiology is considered to have eclampsia. Patients with HELLP syndrome have a form of severe preeclampsia evidenced by thrombocytopenia (maternal platelet count $\leq$ 150,000/μL), hemolysis (microangiopathic hemolytic anemia), and liver dysfunction.

The clinical laboratory tests employed in the evaluation of pregnant women with hypertensive disease are listed in Table 2-1 and described more fully in the subsequent section.

Description of Individual Tests

Hypocalciuria: As early as 17 weeks' gestation, the presence of hypocalciuria ($<$ 195 MgCa+) in a 24-hour urine collection reliably (87%

TABLE 2-1. Hypertensive disease in pregnancy—laboratory testing

Diagnostic and Management Goals	*Tests Used*
1. Screen patients at risk for preeclampsia	24-h urine for calcium Fibronectin
2. Diagnose preeclampsia	Urine for protein Uric acid
3. Detect evidence for HELLP syndrome	Peripheral smear Liver enzymes
4. Differentiate chronic hypertension from preeclampsia	Platelets 24-h urine for calcium
5. Eliminate other causes	Antithrombin III Antinuclear antibody Urinary metanephrines

predictive value) differentiates the patient destined to develop preeclampsia from others in normotensive, gestation hypertensive, and chronically hypertensive categories.

Fibronectin: Circulating plasma concentrations of insoluble cellular fibronectin and total fibronectin increase significantly in patients weeks to months before clinical manifestations of preeclampsia develop. Fibronectin may be one of our best predictors of preeclampsia. The blood level of this marker, however, does not correlate with or predict the later severity of disease nor is it predictive of HELLP syndrome.

Uric Acid: Serum uric acid, one of the oldest and most investigated laboratory tests for the detection of preeclampsia, is an excellent confirmatory test for the presence of preeclampsia, but it is a poor predictor. Elevated serum values correlate well with severe preeclampsia and adverse perinatal outcome.

Proteinuria: Proteinuria is one part of the classic triad of findings that defines preeclampsia. Although it is an excellent reflector of disease severity late in its course, it is not a good predictor. The appearance of proteinuria is associated with a doubling of perinatal mortality.

Liver Function Tests: Alterations in serum concentrations of liver enzymes constitute an inconstant finding in patients with preeclampsia. They increase probably secondary to periportal hemorrhagic necrosis, which may extend to and result in subcapsular hemorrhage or hepatic rupture, particularly in patients with HELLP syndrome. They do, however, accurately reflect the status of disease and recovery in patients with active HELLP syndrome but cannot be used reliably to predict its future development.

Antithrombin III: Antithrombin III activity is depressed in women with preeclampsia/eclampsia and the depression is related to disease severity. The activity remains within a normal range in women with chronic hypertension and decreases only if superimposed preeclampsia is present. Its greatest utility lies in its ability to differentiate chronic hypertension from preeclampsia.

Thrombocytopenia: The most common cause of moderate ($\leq$ 100,000/μL) to severe ($\leq$ 50,000/μL) thrombocytopenia in pregnancy is preeclampsia/eclampsia. Approximately 20% of patients with preeclampsia develop a mild thrombocytopenia (platelet count 100,000–150,000/μL) with little hemostasis risk to the patient or her pregnancy. The severity of HELLP syndrome and the rapidity of recovery is reflected by lactic dehydrogenase and platelet count determinations. The Mississippi classification of HELLP syndrome is based on the lowest peripartal platelet count. In women with preeclampsia and evidence of hemolysis, elevated liver enzymes and thrombocytopenia, a platelet nadir of < 50,000/μL indicates class I HELLP, platelet nadir 50,000/μL–100,000/μL is class II HELLP, and platelet nadir 100,000/μL–150,000/μL is class III HELLP syndrome.

Erythrocyte Morphology, Serum Iron, and Hemoglobin/Hematocrit: Abnormal red cell morphology, increased serum iron, and hemoconcentration individually and collectively sustain a suspected diagnosis of preeclampsia. The extent of their deviation from normal values also reflects preeclampsia severity, but they are poor predictors of the disease.

Miscellaneous: Factor VIII consumption correlates with disease severity in women with preeclampsia, but cannot differentiate these mothers from those with growth-retarded infants, thus limiting its use as a reliable screen for preeclampsia.

Serum prolactin levels have been reported to be elevated or depressed in women with preeclampsia.

β-Thromboglobulin is a good reflector of preeclampsia, but a poor predictor.

Atrial natriuretic peptide cannot differentiate between preeclampsia and chronic hypertension. The complexity of its assay has limited its usefulness in the evaluation of hypertensive disease in pregnancy.

Fibrin degradation products, prothrombin, partial thromboplastin time, and fibrinogen are used in patient management when clinically indicated but are not useful for routine screening studies.

In the future, assays of free and total human chorionic gonadotropin levels and midgestational hyperinsulinemia could assist the clinician to better predict and detect the patient destined to develop hypertensive disease in pregnancy.

References

1. Cunningham FG, MacDonald PC, Gant NF, eds. Hypertensive disorders in pregnancy. In: Williams obstetrics, 18th ed. Norwalk, CT: Appleton & Lange, 1989:653–694.
2. Sibai BM, Anderson GD. Hypertension. In: Gabbe SG, Niebyl JR, Simpson JL, eds. Obstetrics: normal and problem pregnancies, 2d ed. New York: Churchill Livingstone, 1991.

Suggested Reading

Lockwood CJ, Peters JH. Increased plasma levels of ED1+ cellular fibronectin precede the clinical signs of preeclampsia. Am J Obstet Gynecol 1190;162:358–361.

Martin JN, Blake PG, Perry KG, McCaul JF, Hess LW, Martin RW. The natural history of HELLP syndrome: patterns of disease progression and regression. Am J Obstet Gynecol 1991;164:1500–1513.

Martin JN Jr, Stedman CM. Imitators of preeclampsia and HELLP syndrome. In: Cotton DB, ed. Critical care in obstetrics. Obstet Gynecol Clin North Am 1991;18:181–198.

National High Blood Pressure Education Program working group report on high blood pressure in pregnancy. Am J Obstet Gynecol 1990;163:1691–1712.

O'Brien WF. Predicting preeclampsia. Obstet Gynecol 1990;75:445–452.

Sibai BM. Pitfalls in diagnosis and management of preeclampsia. Am J Obstet Gynecol 1988;159:1–5.

3.
Diabetes in Pregnancy

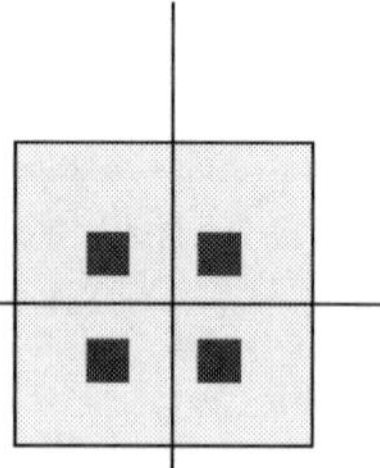

Gerald D. Willett

The clinical laboratory is used extensively in the diagnosis and management of diabetes in pregnancy. The major indications for testing are listed in Table 3-1 and are discussed in more detail in this chapter.

Screening for Diabetes in Pregnancy

The onset or first recognition of carbohydrate intolerance during pregnancy defines gestational diabetes, which is found in 2% to 3% of pregnancies. Some clinicians recommend that all pregnant women undergo screening in pregnancy (1,2). This is usually performed at 24–28 weeks' gestation. If the patient has risk factors (family history, prior stillbirth, age > 30, prior macrosomic infant or one with a malformation, obesity), some clinicians may perform the screen earlier in pregnancy or perform a second screen at 32 weeks if initial testing is negative.

The two-tiered testing regimen recommended in the United States uses an initial nonfasting screening glucose level obtained one hour after a 50-g oral glucose load. Laboratory evaluation, rather than reflectance meter evaluation, is suggested for this screen. If the patient manifests a level of 140 mg/dL or above, she is then scheduled for a 3-hour oral glucose tolerance test (OGTT). Some physicians prefer to use a lower threshold value (130–135 mg/dL) for the initial screening test.

The 3-hour OGTT measures fasting glucose and three hourly levels following a 100-g glucose load. An overnight fast (8–14 hours) is recommended in addition to having the patient consume at least 150 g

---

TABLE 3-1. Indications for testing

1. Screening glucose determinations for the diagnosis of gestational diabetes

2. Glucose testing of the gestational diabetic woman to assess dietary control and need for insulin

3. Preconceptual monitoring of glucose and glycosylated hemoglobin to establish control before pregnancy for the pregestational diabetic patient

4. Laboratory glucose determinations to check reflectance meter results

5. Glycosylated hemoglobin or fructosamine determinations to assess control during pregnancy

6. α-Fetoprotein evaluation for neural tube defects

7. Renal function testing for the pregestational diabetic

8. Pulmonary maturity studies for decisions concerning the timing of delivery

9. Careful monitoring of glucose during labor to avoid neonatal hypoglycemia

10. Postpartum glucose tolerance testing of gestational diabetics

---

carbohydrate daily for 3 days before the test. Some patients do not tolerate the glucose preparation. Reece and colleagues (3) demonstrated acceptable results substituting a glucose polymer for the 100-g glucose preparation. Gestational diabetes is diagnosed if two of the values listed in National Diabetes Data Group (4; Table 3-2) assessment are met or exceeded. These levels have been criticized as representing an overcorrection of the whole blood glucose levels that were used by O'Sullivan and Mahan (5). For this reason, some clinicians use the lower values suggested by Carpenter and Coustan (6; Table 3-2).

Laboratory Management for Gestational Diabetes

Laboratory evaluation of the patient diagnosed with gestational diabetes focuses on the results of dietary management and assessment of need for insulin therapy. Fasting and 2-hour postprandial levels are recommended at weekly intervals. Fasting levels > 105 mg/dL and 2-hour

TABLE 3-2. Glucose tolerance testing

National Diabetes Data Group (two values must be met for diagnosis)

Fasting	105 mg/dL (5.8 mmol/L)
1 h	190 mg/dL (10.6 mmol/L)
2 h	165 mg/dL (9.2 mmol/L)
3 h	145 mg/dL (8.1 mmol/L)

Carpenter and Coustan (two values must be met for diagnosis)

Fasting	95 mg/dL (5.3 mmol/L)
1 h	180 mg/dL (10.0 mmol/L)
2 h	155 mg/dL (8.6 mmol/L)
3 h	140 mg/dL (7.8 mmol/L)

levels > 120 mg/dL signal the need for insulin management. Glucose monitoring for patients requiring β-agonist therapy is important because gestational diabetes is aggravated.

Patients with gestational diabetes who require insulin are instructed in self-monitoring techniques. Periodic comparisons of the patient's reflectance meter glucose levels with clinical laboratory results should be performed. Reflectance meter determinations should be within 10% of the clinical laboratory determinations. Fasting glucose levels plus either preprandial or postprandial measurements should be assessed to guide insulin therapy.

Postpartum Evaluation of Gestational Diabetes

The immediate postpartum evaluation of the woman suspected of gestational diabetes, but who had no evaluation during her pregnancy has proven difficult. Glucose tolerance testing within the first 48 hours following delivery often will not be diagnostic. Carpenter and colleagues (7) measured the sum of incremental change between fasting and both 1-hour and 2-hour determinations. They found that a summed level of 110 mg/dL had more predictive value for antecedent gestational diabetes.

Gestational diabetic women should have a 75-g OGTT performed at the

6-week postpartum visit to evaluate for evidence of diabetes or impaired glucose tolerance. The National Diabetes Data Group criteria for testing is listed in Table 3-3.

Pregestational Diabetes

Establishing good preconception diabetic control with glucose and glycohemoglobin monitoring is important. A number of studies have correlated risk for spontaneous abortions and congenital anomalies with laboratory evidence of poorly controlled diabetes (8–11).

Goals for management of the pregnant insulin-dependent diabetic patient are fasting levels of 60–90 mg/dL, preprandial levels of 60–105 mg/dL, and 2-hour postprandial levels < 120 mg/dL through use of self-monitoring capillary blood glucose techniques. Nocturnal levels may need to be evaluated due to the increased occurrence of nocturnal hypoglycemia in pregnancy.

TABLE 3-3. Postpartum testing of gestational diabetes

National Diabetes Data Group (75-g OGTT)

Diagnostic of diabetes mellitus

1. Fasting glucose levels ≥ 140 mg/dL on two occasions

   or

2. Fasting glucose level < 140 mg/dL but 2-h and one other level (30, 60, 90 min) ≥ 200 mg/dL

   or

3. Symptomatic manifestations of diabetes and random glucose ≥ 200 mg/dL

Diagnostic of impaired glucose tolerance

1. Fasting glucose < 140 mg/dL

   plus

2. 30, 60, or 90-min value during OGTT > 200 mg/dL

   plus

3. Two-hour glucose during OGTT between 140–200 mg/dL

Measurement of urinary ketones by the patient in the morning guards against the development of ketoacidosis and guides her in regard to the adequacy of her previous evening's carbohydrate ingestion. Urinary ketones should be measured whenever the blood glucose value is elevated, particularly during illness.

Additional laboratory testing for insulin-dependent diabetic women includes glycohemoglobin or fructosamine testing to assess diabetic control, maternal serum α-fetoprotein determination to screen for neural tube defects, and renal evaluation in each trimester (urine culture, 24-hour collection for protein and creatinine clearance).

Rarely (and often secondary to an infection) diabetic ketoacidosis (DKA) can occur. Laboratory abnormalities include arterial pH < 7.30, decreased bicarbonate, elevated anion gap, ketonemia, and hyperglycemia. In most cases of DKA the glucose level is > 300, but some cases have occurred with lower levels. Close monitoring of glucose, electrolytes, blood gases, and ketones guides initial insulin and fluid management. With certain laboratory methods the creatinine level may be falsely elevated due to elevated ketones and should be reevaluated once the ketones have cleared.

A principle concern for laboratory assessment during labor is frequent monitoring of glucose to maintain euglycemia and prevent neonatal hypoglycemia. Hourly determinations are made to monitor insulin and fluid replacement with the goal of maintaining glucose in the 70–90 mg/dL range. Postpartum laboratory management is directed toward guiding the patient through the transition when less insulin is needed and protecting against hypoglycemic attacks.

References

1. Cousins L, Baxi L, Chez R, et al. Screening recommendations for gestational diabetes mellitus. Am J Obstet Gynecol 1991;165:493–496.
2. Summary and recommendations of the Second International Workshop-Conference on Gestational Diabetes Mellitus. Diabetes 1985;34(suppl 2): 123–126.
3. Reece EA, Gabrielli S, Abdalla M, O'Connor T, Bargar M, Hobbins JC. Diagnosis of gestational diabetes by use of a glucose polymer. Am J Obstet Gynecol 1989;160:383–384.
4. National Diabetes Data Group. Classification and diagnosis of diabetes mellitus and other categories of glucose intolerance. Diabetes 1979;28:1039–1057.

5. O'Sullivan JB, Mahan CM. Criteria for the oral glucose tolerance test in pregnancy. Diabetes 1964;13:278–285.

6. Carpenter MW, Coustan DR. Criteria for screening tests for gestational diabetes. Am J Obstet Gynecol 1982;144:768–773.

7. Carpenter MW, Coustan DR, Widness JA, Gruppuso PA, Malone M, Rotondo LM. Postpartum testing for antecedent gestational diabetes. Am J Obstet Gynecol 1988;159:1128–1131.

8. Miller E, Hare JW, Cloherty JP, et al. Elevated maternal hemoglobin A1c in early pregnancy and major congenital anomalies in infants of diabetic mothers. N Engl J Med 1981;304:1331–1334.

9. Rosenn B, Miodovnik M, Dignan PS, Siddiqi TA, Khoury J, Mimouni F. Minor congenital malformations in infants of insulin-dependent diabetic women: association with poor glycemic control. Obstet Gynecol 1990;76: 745–749.

10. Rosenn B, Miodovnik M, Combs CA, Khoury J, Siddiqi TA. Pre-conception management of insulin-dependent diabetes: improvement of pregnancy outcome. Obstet Gynecol 1991;77:846–849.

11. Kitzmiller JL, Gavin LA, Gin GD, Jovanovic-Peterson L, Main EK, Sigrang WD. Preconception care of diabetes. JAMA 1991;6:731–736.

Suggested Reading

Amon E, Lipshitz J, Sibai B, Abdella TN, Whybrew DW, el-Nazer A. Quantitative analysis of amniotic fluid phospholipids in diabetic pregnant women. Obstet Gynecol 1986;68:373.

Blumenthal SA, Abdul-Karim RW. Diagnosis, classification, and metabolic management of diabetes in pregnancy: therapeutic impact of self-monitoring of blood glucose and of newer methods of insulin delivery. Obstet Gynecol Surv 1987;42:593–604.

Greene MF, Benacerraf BR. Prenatal diagnosis in diabetic gravidas: utility of ultrasound and maternal serum alpha-fetoprotein screening. Obstet Gynecol 1991;77:520–524.

Harkness LJ, Ashwood ER, Parsons S, Lenke RR. Comparison of the accuracy of glucose reflectance meters in pregnant insulin-dependent diabetics. Obstet Gynecol 1991;77:181–185.

Kitzmiller JL, Brown ER, Phillippe M, et al. Diabetic nephropathy and perinatal outcome. Am J Obstet Gynecol 1981;141:741.

Kjos SL, Walther FJ, Montoro M, Paul RH, Diaz F, Stabler M. Prevalence and etiology of respiratory distress in infants of diabetic mothers: predictive value of fetal lung maturation tests. Am J Obstet Gynecol 1990;163:898–903.

Milunsky A, Alpert E, Kitzmiller JL, Younger MD, Neff RK. Prenatal diagnosis of neural tube defects; VIII. The importance of serum alpha-fetoprotein screening in diabetic women. Am J Obstet Gynecol 1982;142:1030–1032.

Nesler CL, Sinclair SH, Schwartz SS, Gabbe SG. Diabetic nephropathy in pregnancy. Clin Obstet Gynecol 1985;28:528–535.

Reece EA, Coustan DR, Hayslett JP, et al. Diabetic nephropathy: pregnancy performance and fetomaternal outcome. Am J Obstet Gynecol 1988;159:56–66.

4.
Viral Infections

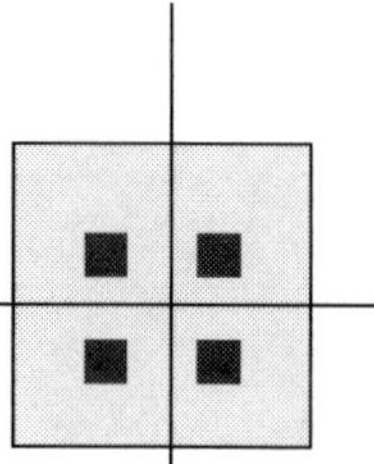

Periclis Roussis
Berry A. Campbell
Susan M. Cox

This chapter discusses the clinical laboratory evaluation for viral ill-
nesses commonly encountered by the obstetrician-gynecologist. Specimen
collection and notes on laboratory testing of specific viral infections
(cytomegalovirus [CMV], herpes simplex [HSV], varicella-zoster [VZV],
rubella, the hepatitis viruses, and human immunodeficiency virus [HIV])
are included in addition to a table illustrating common test methodologies
(Table 4-1). Additional information for these viruses and others (papillomavirus, coxsackie, and parvovirus) can also be found in Part 7.

Specimen Collection

Selection of appropriate specimens for the detection of viral infections is
critical in addition to obtaining an adequate sample. Aspirates, scrapings,
and tissue specimens are generally preferred over swab specimens if available. Cultures should be obtained during the first week of illness because
the viral yield rapidly decreases after the fourth day of infection. Each
specimen should be accompanied by serum (acute titer) with a convalescent serum obtained 2–3 weeks later.

Specimens should be collected in sterile containers to prevent bacterial
or fungal contamination and submitted to the laboratory as rapidly as
possible. Several types of commercially available transport media are suit-
able for viral specimens. In situations where transport media are not available, sterile swabs may be placed in a tube of buffered bacterial broth.
Specimens should be processed as quickly as possible. If a delay of 1–5

TABLE 4-1. Viral testing methodologies

Cell Culture

"Gold standard" method. Inoculation of viable virus into cell culture. Initial interpretation based on identification of cytopathic effects. Immunologic assays performed on monolayers or supernatant are used for confirmation of results. Results are obtained in a few days to several weeks.

Spin Amplification Cell Culture (shell vial method)

Variation of conventional culture. Centrifugation increases infectivity of certain viruses for cell monolayer. Results obtained sooner (24–72 h)

Electron Microscopy (EM)

Identification is based on morphology and size. For EM to be useful, the titer of virus must be at least 10^6 to 10^7 particles/mL. Rarely performed for clinical testing.

Immunologic Assays

These methods rely on the ability of virus-specific antibodies to bind to viral antigens. The virus does not need to be viable but antigenicity must be preserved. Rapid results possible with high degree of sensitivity and specificity. Examples of immunologic assays include: counter immunoelectrophoresis, direct and indirect immunofluorescence, immunoperoxidase methods, radioimmunoassay, enzyme immunoassay, and latex agglutination.

Nucleic Acid Probes

Specific viral nucleic acid may be detected either in tissue or in cell cultures by hybridization technology. To increase sensitivity, polymerase chain reaction is used.

Serologic Tests

These tests detect and quantitate virus specific antibody in a patient's serum. Methods include:

Complement fixation (CF): Serial dilutions of the patient's serum are incubated with viral antigen and known amount of complement. If antibodies in the serum react with the virus, the complement will be fixed and consumed. The CF antibodies are primarily IgG and typically develop during the convalescent state, thus the test is commonly used in evaluating acute and convalescent titers.

TABLE 4-1, continued

Neutralizing antibodies test: This test measures the ability of the patient's serum to block cell culture infectivity by a standard inoculum of a specific virus. If the virus in not neutralized, its presence may be detected by cytopathic effects. Time consuming.

Hemagglutination inhibition test: Some viruses have hemagglutinins, which are antigens capable of clumping erythrocytes of certain species. Inhibition of the clumping reaction by virus-specific antibodies in the patient's serum is the basis for the test.

Immunofluorescence: Serial dilutions of the patient's serum are reacted with viral antigens fixed on a slide. Detection is by a fluorescein-conjugated antibody specific for human immunoglobulin.

Western blot (immunoblot): This technique combines electrophoresis and blotting methodologies. The clinician is most familiar with use of this test in the diagnosis of HIV. Here the test is performed by exposure of electrophoretically separated viral components to patient sera. The proteins in the HIV core and envelope are isolated by gel electrophoresis, transferred to paper, and antibody is detected by enzymatic reaction. Positive sera will react with the viral core proteins or envelope proteins; negative sera are nonreactive.

days is anticipated, specimens should be stored and transported at 4°C rather than frozen. If specimens are expected to be in transit longer than 5 days, they should be frozen at $-70°C$ initially and shipped on dry ice. Viral specimens should never be stored or transported at $-20°C$.

Cytomegalovirus

Recognized as the most common cause of intrauterine infection, CMV infects 1% to 2% of all newborns in the United States. Laboratory testing for CMV is usually performed in situations of maternal symptoms or when sonographic abnormalities are discovered consistent with fetal infection (see Chapter 9). Evidence of maternal infection can be obtained through culture (urine, blood, saliva, cervical secretions) and serology. Fetal infection can be established from amniotic fluid and fetal blood studies. Spin amplification techniques have allowed a more rapid culture determination (sometimes within 24 hours). Cordocentesis allows for evaluation of anemia, thrombocytopenia, altered liver enzymes, and total immunoglobulin in addition to viral culture and CMV-IgM. Determining pregnancy management on the basis of CMV laboratory results alone remains problematic because testing does not predict well which infants will develop significant problems. Routine serologic screening of pregnant patients or patients before conception has limited value because many infected infants develop normally and no vaccine is available.

Herpes Simplex

Testing for HSV is performed on patients initially presenting with symptoms of painful genital ulcerations. The highest culture recovery rates are obtained from aspirating or swabbing new vesicular lesions. Spin amplification techniques can reduce culture times. Direct examination of slide preparations stained with Giemsa, hematoxylin and eosin, Wright, or Papanicolaou stains can be used to identify ground glass multinuclear change and inclusions. Serologic evaluation of patients is seldom indicated, but it may rarely be useful in documenting a true primary infection (fourfold increase in titer, acute to convalescent). IgM antibody may persist for about 8 weeks following primary infection. Serologic identification of recurrence, infection with a new herpes type virus, and separation of HSV-1 from HSV-2 is difficult with the present commercially available assays.

Laboratory evaluation of pregnant patients is generally confined to the initial confirmation of HSV if lesions appear during pregnancy. Serial weekly cultures for HSV are not necessary nor is amniocentesis recommended to diagnose fetal infection. Lesion identification and assessment for prodromal symptoms are used in making a decision regarding mode of delivery.

Varicella-Zoster Virus

Similar to HSV, VZV can be identified through analysis of vesicle fluid or material swabbed from the base of fresh lesions. Fluorescent assays using a monoclonal antibody can identify VZV in less than an hour. The most frequent use of serology is to determine if a woman exposed to VZV is immune and thus not a candidate for immunoglobulin administration. Several assays are available for assessment of VZV infection, but the enzyme-linked immunosorbent assay (ELISA) is often used due to its good correlation with neutralizing antibody titer and ease of performance. Serologic diagnosis of recent infection requires a fourfold or greater rise in antibody titer.

Rubella

Rubella antibody testing is routinely performed to establish the immune status of patients. To document immunity, the patient should be tested for the presence of IgG-specific rubella antibody. An individual with a hemagglutination inhibition titer $\geq$ 1:8 is considered immune.

Rubella antibody levels are depicted in Figure 4-1. The following points must be kept in mind when evaluating a patient for possible rubella exposure:

1. Significant elevation of IgM indicates acute rubella.
2. If recent exposure (one week) and IgM are negative, repeat in 2–3 weeks; if still negative, acute rubella is excluded.
3. If recent exposure and initial IgG are negative, repeat in 2–3 weeks. If it undergoes a fourfold increase in titer, then acute rubella is diagnosed.
4. If IgG has a detectable titer and then undergoes a fourfold increase in 2–3 weeks, the patient may have either acute rubella or an acute stage of rubella *reinfection*.
5. Because of the promptness of the antibody response, it is important to get serologic studies as soon as possible after the exposure or development of the rash. If testing is delayed following exposure or onset of symptoms, IgG and IgM testing should still be performed. Rising titers of IgG or significant elevations of IgM may still be able to diagnose an acute infection.

Hepatitis Viruses

Laboratory testing for hepatitis is performed in prenatal examinations and in patients developing jaundice. The primary test used in prenatal screening is the test for hepatitis B surface antigen (HBsAg). Figure 4-2 illustrates the laboratory studies for hepatitis A (HAV) and B (HBV) used in the evaluation of the jaundiced patient.

Tests for HAV antigen are not available. Diagnosis is based on two types of antibody to hepatitis A (IgM or IgG). As shown in Figure 4-3, the interpretation of HAV antibody results depends on the time the specimen was obtained relative to onset of clinical symptoms. IgM positivity or a rising IgG is indicative of infection.

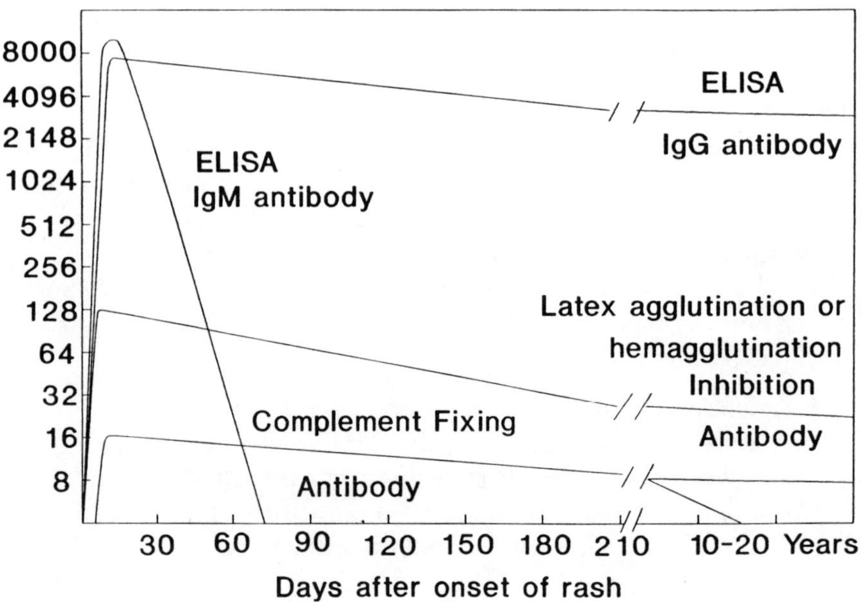

FIGURE 4-1. Rubella antibody levels.

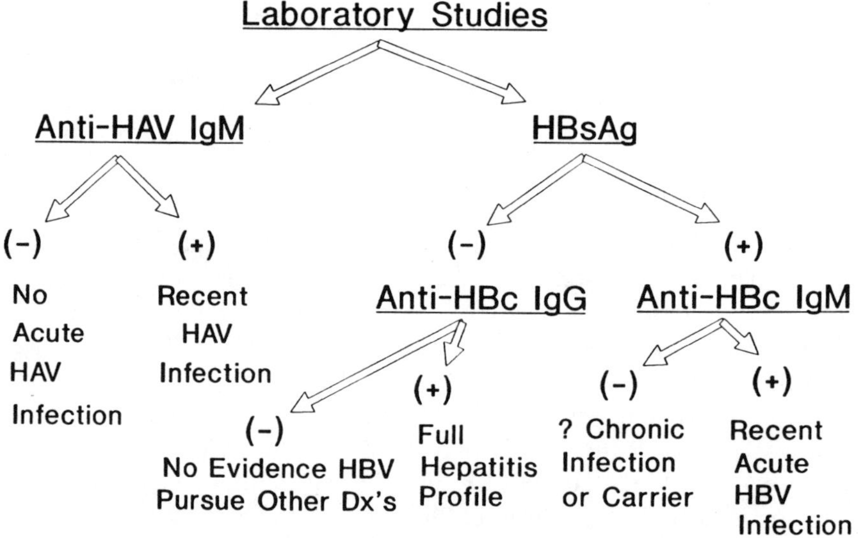

FIGURE 4-2. Recommended work-up of a jaundiced patient.

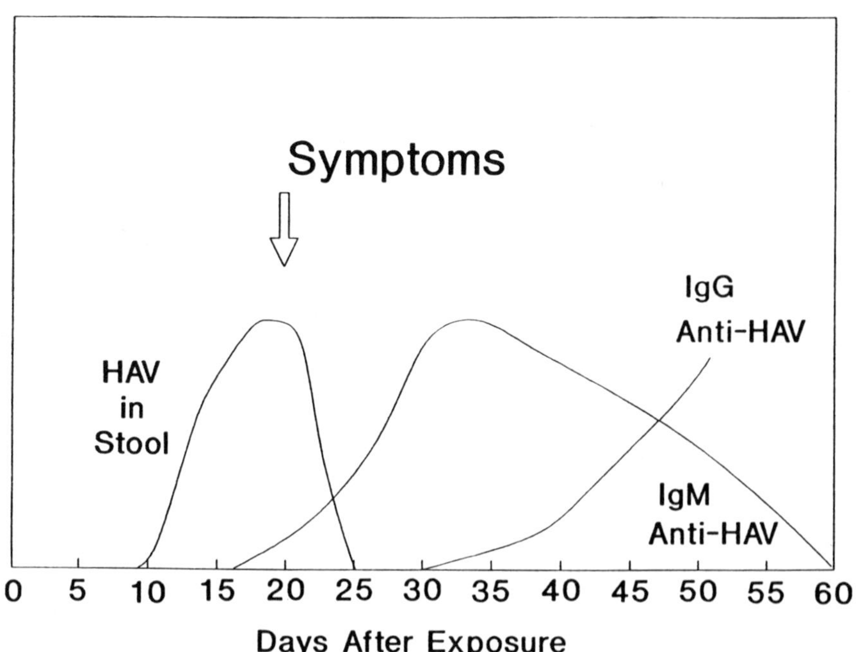

FIGURE 4-3. Antibody response in HAV infections.

Prenatal screening for HBsAg is important because HBV traverses the placenta and therefore congenital fetal exposure is possible. A number of antigen and antibody tests are used for evaluation of hepatitis B. These are described in Part 7.

Perinatal transmission of hepatitis C has been reported. Prenatal screening for hepatitis C should be performed in patients at high risk (intravenous drug use, sexually promiscuous, history of acute hepatitis of unknown etiology). All positive hepatitis C screening tests should be confirmed by the newer more specific recombinant immunoblot assay.

Human Immunodeficiency Virus

Testing for HIV should be offered to pregnant patients or those contemplating pregnancy. Testing should be discussed with all gynecologic patients at risk. Initial laboratory testing for HIV is performed with ELISA. False positive ELISAs have been seen in patients with autoimmune disease, lymphoproliferative disorders, multiparity, and in people who have received multiple blood transfusions. Positive screening assays require confirmation by Western blot.

Western blot analyzes antibodies in the patient's serum to a number of electrophoretically separated HIV proteins and glycoproteins. Sera from definitely infected individuals show variable reactivity with the HIV proteins on Western blot. Unfortunately, different criteria for a positive test have been established. Slightly different criteria have been established by the Department of Defense, the American Red Cross, and the Food and Drug Administration (FDA). Strips that do not meet criteria but show some reaction are termed indeterminate. Approximately 15% of sera from noninfected persons tested by the FDA-licensed Western blot (Du-Pont) show this indeterminate pattern. The significance of an indeterminate blot is at present poorly understood.

Suggested Reading

American College of Obstetricians and Gynecologists. Human immunodeficiency virus infections. Technical Bulletin no. 169, June 1992.

American College of Obstetricians and Gynecologists. Perinatal herpes simplex virus infections. Technical Bulletin no. 122, November 1988.

Bryan JA. The serologic diagnosis of viral infection. Arch Pathol Lab Med 1987;111:1015–1023.

Hermann KL. Available rubella serologic tests. Rev Infect Dis 1985;7(suppl): 108–112.

Hollinger FB. Serologic evaluation of viral hepatitis. Hosp Pract 1987;22(2): 101–114.

Leland DS, French MLV. Virus isolation and identification. In: Lennette EH, Halonen P, Murphy FA, eds. Laboratory diagnosis of infectious diseases: principles and practice. New York: Springer-Verlag, 1988.

Schmidt NJ, Emmons RW, eds. Diagnostic procedures for viral, rickettsial, and chlamydial infections. Washington DC: American Public Health Association, Inc, 1989.

Sever J. Infections in pregnancy: highlights from the collaborative perinatal project. Teratology 1982;25:227–237.

Tony MJ, Thursby M, Rakela J, et al. Studies on the maternal-infant transmission of viruses which cause acute hepatitis. Gastroenterology 1981;80:999–1004.

5.
Bacterial Infections

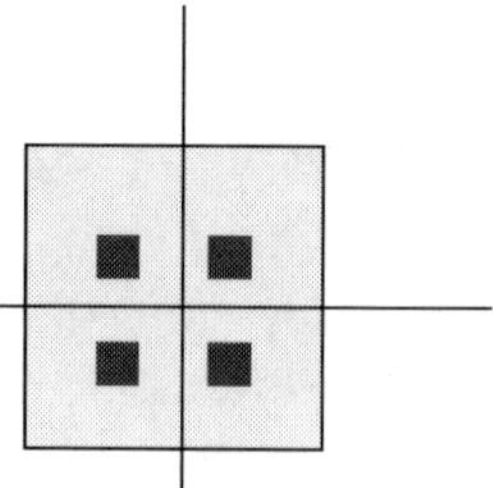

Susan Marie Mou

This chapter focuses on the clinical laboratory evaluation of specific bacterial infections in pregnancy, intra-amniotic infections, postpartum endometritis, and urinary tract infections in pregnancy.

Gonococcus in Pregnancy

Disseminated gonococcal infections (DGI) are more common in pregnancy (1,2). Forty percent of DGI cases are in pregnancy or the puerperium. Blood culture for gonococcus is the best method of detection. Cervical, rectal, and pharyngeal cultures may be necessary, depending on patient history of exposure sites.

Neisseria gonorrhoeae is a relatively fastidious organism, and the culture should be obtained, transported, and plated as soon as possible. Transport devices, using selective growth media and self-generating carbon dioxide, are the time-honored standards for diagnosis of genital gonorrhea. Gram stains from cervical smears have a sensitivity of only 40% to 50% at best (3) and are not adequate for clinical use. Enzyme-linked immunosorbent assays (ELISA) and immunofluorescence tests for gonorrhea lack sensitivity. An immunofluorescent test using a monoclonal antibody offers greater specificity, but may limit the number of strains of *N gonorrhoeae* that will be detected. The DNA probes recently developed can detect *N gonorrhoeae* in as little as 2 hours (4–6). They are as sensitive and specific as culture and are advantageous because of rapid turnaround time.

Chlamydia in Pregnancy

The role of chlamydial infection in pregnancy remains controversial. Chlamydia infections have been linked to premature rupture of membranes (PROM), preterm labor, low birthweight, and stillbirth. Vertical transmission is documented, with conjunctivitis and pneumonitis in newborns. Postabortal, postcesarean section and postpartum maternal infections may also be associated with chlamydia.

In pregnant, as in nonpregnant women, cervical chlamydia cultures are 100% specific and 80% to 90% sensitive (7). Direct fluorescent antibody and enzyme immunoassay tests have high specificity and sensitivity in high prevalence populations. However, in groups of women with lower prevalences, culture techniques are more accurate (8). Nucleic acid probes have a 98.4% correlation with culture in asymptomatic pregnant women (9). When obtaining specimens, it must be remembered that endocervical cells are required for an adequate specimen, and among the rapid screens, direct fluorescent antibody testing is the only one that tells the practitioner of the adequacy of the specimen. Only culture is applicable to all anatomic sites and specimens. Current recommendations of the Centers for Disease Control and Prevention for screening asymptomatic pregnant women for *Chlamydia trachomatis* are listed in Table 5-1.

Intra-amniotic Infections

The majority of intra-amniotic infections occur in women with ruptured membranes, but infection may also occur with intact membranes. A number of different organisms have been reported with intra-amniotic infection. These include *Bacteroides* species, group B streptococci, *Escherichia coli* and other gram-negative rods, *Clostridium* species, *Peptococcus* species, and *Listeria monocytogenes*.

Amniocentesis may be used to obtain specimens for aerobic and anaerobic culture. Alternatively, if membranes are ruptured, a culture can be obtained by transcervical aspirate, aspirating 3–5 mL intrauterine catheter fluid, discarding it, and then sending the next 2–3 mL for culture. Gram stain results need to be interpreted with caution—finding no leukocytes or bacteria excludes intra-amniotic infection, but the presence of leukocytes may be normal in labor. If listeria is suspected, notify the laboratory so that listeria can be distinguished from diptheroids.

Recent work by Romero and colleagues (10) shows that an amniotic fluid

TABLE 5-1. Centers for Disease Control and Prevention recommendations for screening and treatment of maternal *C trachomatis* infection in pregnant women

A. Who?
Pregnant women should undergo diagnostic tests* for:
 C trachomatis
 N gonorrhoeae
 Syphilis

B. When?
Initial visit and again in third trimester if judged at increased risk, ie, < 25 yr of age, history of sexually transmitted disease, new (< 3 mo) sexual partner or multiple partners

C. Recommended regimens[†,‡]
Oral erythromycin base, 500 mg q.i.d. for 7 d
 If poorly tolerated:
Oral erythromycin base, 250 mg q.i.d. for 14 d
 or
Oral amoxicillin, 500 mg t.i.d. for 7 d

D. Partner
Evaluate and treat if contact within 30 d; if tests unavailable, treat

E. How?
Tests of cure (by culture) are not recommended unless there is question of patient compliance

Modified from Centers for Disease Control. 1989 Sexually transmitted disease treatment guidelines. MMWR 1989;38(suppl 8):27–28.

*See text
[†]Poor tolerance is treated with supportive care or use alternative regimen
[‡]Enteric-coated or sustained-release preparations of erythromycin are also effective but more costly

white blood cell count of $\geq$ 50 cells/mm^3, obtained by transabdominal amniocentesis in women with preterm labor and intact fetal membranes, is associated with intra-amniotic infections. The amniotic fluid was examined in the hematology laboratory with a hemocytometer, the absolute white cell count calculated by multiplying the area examined by a factor of 10 per area and expressed as number of cells per mm^3. This quick screening may be helpful in managing women with intra-amniotic infection. Cultures may take days to grow.

Culturing of fetal membranes between the amnion and chorion with sterile Dacron swabs (11) and subsequent examination of the placenta, umbilical cord, and membranes by pathology are two tools useful after delivery in determining possible infectious etiologies associated with birth.

Urinary Tract Infections in Pregnancy

Asymptomatic bacteriuria occurs in 2% to 7% of pregnant women. Indigent women, those with sickle cell trait, and diabetic women have higher prevalences (12). If asymptomatic bacteriuria is not treated, one third of these women develop acute pyelonephritis during pregnancy (13). Urine cultures show significant bacteriuria if at least 100,000 colonies/mL can be grown from a freshly voided midstream urine that has been in the bladder for 2 hours. Stamm and colleagues have shown that lower colony counts of 20,000 or more may be associated with active infection in symptomatic women (14). Routine urine cultures of populations of pregnant women with high risk of asymptomatic bacteriuria should be performed at the initial obstetric visit and the patients treated with appropriate antibiotics.

Acute pyelonephritis will still complicate 1% to 2% of pregnancies. Urinalysis will microscopically detect bacteria. Urine cultures with sensitivities isolate the infective organism and help to tailor antibiotic regimens. Blood cultures, serum electrolytes, serum creatinine, and complete blood count should also be performed. The serum creatinine may rise and anemia develop due to endotoxin lipopolysaccharide damage to peritubular capillaries (15) and red blood cells, respectively (16). Similarly, endotoxin may cause acute respiratory distress syndrome, diagnosed by chest radiograph, tachypnea, and abnormal blood gases. Endotoxins may also cause septic shock, which is uncommon and is diagnosed clinically.

Postpartum Endomyometritis

The diagnosis of postpartum endomyometritis is usually based on clinical findings, including fever, abdominal pain and tenderness, malaise, foul lochia, and increased white cell count. Cultures to be sent include intrauterine cultures and venous blood cultures, both aerobic and anaerobic. A double-lumen or triple-lumen catheter (17) or a povidone-iodine cleansed, dilated cervix through which a cotton swab is passed (18) avoids bacterial contamination by vaginal flora when you are obtaining aerobic and anaerobic transcervical uterine cultures. However, many microbiology laboratories will not plate endocervically obtained anaerobic endometrial cultures, and you need to first inform the laboratory if you intend to use a technique that avoids vaginal contamination so that the lab will plate anaerobic cultures. Urine culture and urinalysis may also help rule out a urinary tract infection as the cause of infectious morbidity, as will a sputum Gram stain and culture in women with pulmonary findings. Gram stains of uterine specimens are helpful only when sheets of hemolytic streptococci, clostridia, or other anaerobes are present. In women who do not respond to antibiotics in 48–72 hours, repeat the pelvic examination and complete blood count. Ultrasound is helpful in diagnosing retained products of conception and septic pelvic thrombophlebitis (19). Computed tomography scans (20) and magnetic resonance imaging may also delineate pelvic thrombophlebitis.

Syphilis in Pregnancy

Syphilis is associated with premature birth, stillbirths, congenital anomalies, and neonatal morbidity and mortality. Absolute diagnosis in women can be made by identifying *Treponema pallidum* with darkfield examination of fresh moist chancre scrapings or secondary syphilis lesions. More frequently patients are asymptomatic and nontreponemal tests such as rapid plasma reagin and VDRL should be drawn at least at the first prenatal visit and again in the third trimester. These serology tests may be falsely reactive in a variety of maternal conditions, thus a confirmatory fluorescent treponemal antibody absorption test or microhemagglutination assay for antibodies to *T pallidum* should be performed. Amniotic fluid studies (darkfield and immunofluorescence) have been used to identify evidence of congenital syphilis (21,22).

References

1. Al-Suleiman SA, Grimes EM, Jonas HS. Disseminated gonococcal infections. Obstet Gynecol 1983;61:48–51.
2. Holmes KK, Counts GW, Beaty HN. Disseminated gonococcal infection. Ann Intern Med 1971;74:979–993.
3. Ison C. Methods of diagnosing gonorrhea. Genitourin Med 1990;66:453–459.
4. Granato P, Franz MR. Use of the Gen-Probe PACE system for the detection of

Neisseria gonorrhoeae in urogenital samples. Diag Microbiol Infect Dis 1990;13:217–221.

5. Panke E, Yang L, Leist P, Magevney P, Fry R, Lee R. Comparison of Gen-Probe DNA probe test and culture for the detection of *Neisseria gonorrhoeae* in endocervical specimens. J Clin Microbiol 1991;29:883–888.

6. Granato P, Franz MR. Evaluation of a protype DNA probe test for the noncultural diagnosis of gonorrhea. J Clin Microbiol 1989;27:632–635.

7. Barnes RC. Laboratory diagnosis of human chlamydial infections. Clin Microbiol Rev 1989;2:119–136.

8. McGregor JA, French JI. *Chlamydia trachomatis* infection during pregnancy. Am J Obstet Gynecol 1991;164:1782–1789.

9. Yang LI, Panke ES, Leist PA, Fry RJ, Lee RF. Detection of *Chlamydia trachomatis* endocervical infection in asymptomatic and symptomatic women: comparison of deoxyribonucleic acid probe test with tissue culture. Am J Obstet Gynecol 1991;165:1444–1453.

10. Romero R, Quintero R, Nores J, et al. Amniotic fluid white blood cell count: a rapid and simple test to diagnose microbial invasion of the amniotic cavity and predict preterm delivery. Am J Obstet Gynecol 1991;165:821–830.

11. Hillier SL, Martius J, Krohn MA, Kiviat NB, Holmes KK, Eschenbach DA. A case-control study of chorioamniotic infection and histologic chorioamnionitis in prematurity. N Engl J Med 1988;319:972–978.

12. Cunningham FG. Acute pyelonephritis complicating pregnancy. In: Williams obstetrics, 17th ed., suppl 18. June/July, 1988.

13. Whalley PJ. Bacteriuria of pregnancy. Am J Obstet Gynecol 1967;97:723–738.

14. Stamm WE, Counts GW, Running KR, Fihn S, Turck M, Holmes KK. Diagnosis of coliform infection in acutely dysuric women. N Engl J Med 1982;307:463–468.

15. Richman AV, Gerber LI, Balis JU. Peritubular capillaries: a major target site of endotoxin-induced vascular injury. Lab Invest 1980;43:327–332.

16. Cox S, Shelburne P, Mason RA, Cunningham FG. Erythrocyte morphology in women with acute pyelonephritis. (abstract). Presented at the Infectious Disease Society for Obstetrics-Gynecology, Aspen, Colo., August 1988.

17. Rosene K, Eschenbach DA, Tompkins LS, et al. Polymicrobial early postpartum endometritis with facultative and anaerobic bacterial genital mycoplasmas and *C. trachomatis:* treatment with piperacillin or cefoxitin. J Infect Dis 1986;153:1028–1037.

18. Martens MG, Faro S, Hammill H, Phillips LE, Riddle GD. Comparison of two endometrial sampling devices, cotton-tipped swab and double-lumen catheter with a brush. J Reprod Med 1989;34:875–879.

19. Faustin D, Minkoff H, Schaffer R, et al. Relationship of ultrasound find-

ings after cesarean section to operative morbidity. Obstet Gynecol 1985;
66:195–198.

20. Brown CEL, Lowe TW, Cunningham FG, et al. Puerperal pelvic thrombophlebitis: impact on diagnosis and treatment using x-ray computed tomography and magnetic resonance imaging. Obstet Gynecol 1986;68:789–794.

21. Wendel GD, Maberry MC, Christmas JT, Goldberg MS, Norgard MV. Examination of amniotic fluid in diagnosing congenital syphilis with fetal death.
Obstet Gynecol 1989;74:687–693.

22. Wendel GD, Sanchez PJ, Peters MT, Harstad TW, Potter LL, Norgard MV.
Identification of *Treponema pallidum* in amniotic fluid and fetal blood from
pregnancies complicated by congenital syphilis. Obstet Gynecol 1991;78:
890–894.

6.

Fungal and Parasitic Infections

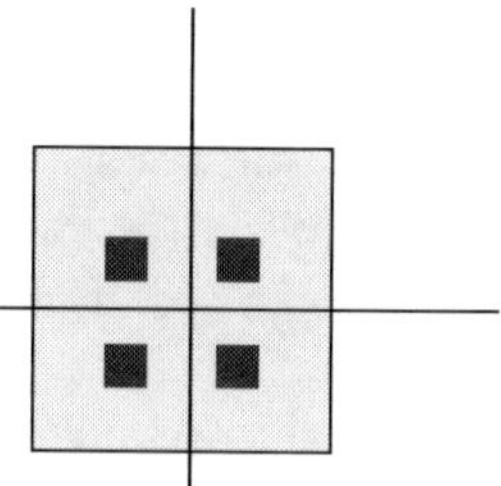

Susan Marie Mou

Fungal and parasitic infections in pregnancy have received increased attention because of the emergence of human immunodeficiency virus (HIV) infections, an increase in numbers of organ transplant patients, and an increase in the at risk immigrant populations. A general listing of pertinent organisms along with laboratory testing is found in Tables 6-1 and 6-2. This chapter provides clinical and laboratory information on infections secondary to *Candida* species, *Cryptococcus neoformans, Toxoplasma gondii, Giardia lamblia, Entamoeba histolytica, Pneumocystis carinii, Trichinella spiralis,* and schistosomiasis. Additional information can also be obtained in Part 7.

Candida Infections

Candida species can be isolated from the vagina in 30% of pregnant women (1–3). Few cases of candidal sepsis have been reported. Immuno-suppressed patients, both those with organ transplants and with diseases such as HIV infection, and women with foreign bodies such as intrauterine devices, catheters, and cervical cerclage may encounter more problems with systemic disease. Data on 8 pregnant women with symptomatic can-didemia have been described (4).

Infants can have antenatal candidal chorioamnionitis and funisitis. When candida is suspected or there is neonatal or maternal sepsis of unclear etiology, cultures can be obtained from pathology specimens, blood, vagina, and localized sites of infection (ie, cerebrospinal fluid,

TABLE 6-1. Laboratory testing for fungal diseases

Fungal Diseases	*Laboratory Tests*
Candidal infection	Vaginal smear (KOH) Culture (vagina, mouth, blood) PAS, silver stains (placental tissue)
Histoplasmosis	Culture (sputum, blood) Serology (immunodiffusion, complement fixation, radioimmunoassay) Bone marrow (staining and culture)
Coccidioidomycosis	Skin testing Serology (latex agglutination and immunodiffusion techniques)
Aspergillosis	Culture (from infected sites)
Cryptococcosis	Microscopic exam of infected tissue Culture (infected tissue, blood) Antigen titers

mouth). When candidemia is suspected, specific culture techniques such as lysis centrifugation may also be helpful (5). Placental involvement includes the umbilical cord, extraplacental membranes, chorionic surface, and rarely the intervillous space and chorionic villi. Periodic acid-Schiff or Gomori methenamine silver stains of pathology specimens are more sensitive than routine hemotoxylin and eosin staining for detecting *Candida* species (6).

Cryptococcosis

Cryptococcus neoformans is an important pathogen in immunocompromised hosts. It occurs in 6% to 10% of patients with acquired immunodeficiency syndrome (AIDS) in the United States. Ninety percent of patients with AIDS who are infected with *C neoformans* develop meningitis. However, cryptococcal infection has also been described in the lung, liver, skin, lymph nodes, adrenal glands, and many other organs. Microscopic colonies-encapsulated budding yeasts can be seen in infected tissues. Cryptococcosis of the placenta has been described in a woman with AIDS. The infant was not affected. Cryptococcus organisms

TABLE 6-2. Laboratory testing for parasitic diseases

Parasitic Disease	*Laboratory Testing*
Toxoplasmosis	Serology (maternal and fetal blood) Culture (fetal blood or amniotic fluid) Experimental: Polymerase chain reaction technique
Malaria	Peripheral blood smear Indirect fluorescent antibody
Giardiasis	Stool examination Small bowel aspirate
Amebiasis	Stool examination Sigmoid exudate evaluation Serology
Chagas' disease	Direct examination of blood Serology Xenodiagnosis
Trichomoniasis	Vaginal wet smear Culture
Cryptosporidiosis	Stool examination Endoscopic biopsy
Pneumocystosis	Microscopic evaluation of sputum, bronchial washing, or transbronchial specimens
Helminthic infections	Many of these infections are intestinal (evaluation of stool and other gastrointestinal specimens) Complete blood counts may reveal anemia and eosinophilia Serum proteins may be decreased Serologic testing may be helpful in some of the diseases (trichinosis, filariasis)

can be also be identified by Grocott's modification of Gomori methenamine silver and mucicarmine stains (7). Blood cultures as well as cultures from infected tissues may grow out cryptococcus. Cryptococcal antigen titers can also be performed to help in diagnosis (8).

Toxoplasmosis

Toxoplasma gondii is an important obstetric infection. Infection occurs after ingestion of material contaminated by cat feces or ingestion of tissue cysts in undercooked meat. Prevention of infection in pregnancy is the key element in preventing toxoplasmosis in the United States. One of a thousand infants born in the United States demonstrates congenital toxoplasmosis (9). Intrauterine infection is possible only when women have active toxoplasmosis with circulating tachyzoites, primarily nonimmune mothers with their first infection, and rarely in latently infected immunocompromised mothers experiencing reactivation of their disease. Diagnosis is difficult. Positive serology by the Sabin-Feldman dye test or indirect immunofluorescent antibody (IFA) testing may be quantitated so that rising titers are demonstrated. The IgG and sometimes IgM-IFA titers may remain positive for years. The double sandwich IgM enzyme-linked immunosorbent assay (ELISA) has greater sensitivity and specificity than the IgM-IFA. In one study 93% of individuals with recent infection were positive by IgM-ELISA, but negative by IgM-IFA. In congenital toxoplasmosis, positive IgM-ELISA occurs in 73% of mothers versus positive IgM-IFA in 25%. Isolation of toxoplasmosis in tissue culture or mice culture from cordocentesis specimens of fetal blood or amniotic fluid should also be performed if infection is suspected; this remains the most definitive diagnostic technique. IgM titers may be performed on fetal blood, but false positives due to maternal-fetal hemorrhage and rheumatoid factor-containing sera, and false negatives limit the interpretation of IgM in cord blood. Polymerase chain reaction techniques on amniotic fluid may soon replace all other testing.

Giardiasis

Giardiasis is caused by *G lamblia*. It is the most commonly identified pathogenic intestinal parasite in the United States (10). Giardiasis may range from asymptomatic to severe diarrhea with malabsorption. Patients may have explosive, watery, foul-smelling, bulky, diarrhea; abdominal cramps; nausea; low-grade fever; chills; and malaise. Fresh stool samples will fail to demonstrate blood or mucus. Early in the infection, trophozoites are found in the stool. Later, cyst forms are found in more formed stools. Duodenal aspirate demonstrates trophozoites. Generally, giardiasis has minimal effects on pregnancy; however, malabsorption accompanied by weight loss and debility may impair fertility and adversely affect the pregnancy.

Amebiasis

Amebiasis can be more severe and have a higher fatality rate in pregnant women. Amebiasis is caused by ingestion of the cyst form of *E histolytica* and then trophozoite multiplication in the colon. The pregnant patient may be asymptomatic or may have fulminate dysentery. Pregnancy, immunosuppression, malnutrition, and steroid therapy may result in clinical disease. Diagnosis is made by observation of trophozoite or cyst forms in fresh stool. Sigmoidoscopy shows punctate hemorrhagic areas or small exudative ulcers with hyperemic borders. Exudative material from the ulcerations may help in the diagnosis along with serologic studies.

Pneumocystosis

Pneumocystis carinii is unclassified but is considered to be a protozoan parasite. It is an important pathogen in immunocompromised patients. Maternal deaths have been reported in pregnant AIDS patients with *P carinii* pneumonia. In symptomatic patients with progressive cough, shortness of breath, and fever, variable chest x-ray abnormalities may be seen; diagnosis is made by finding the organism in sputum, bronchial washing, or transbronchial biopsy specimens. These fluids are stained with Giemsa or silver methanamine (11).

Trichinosis

Infection with *T spiralis* is caused by ingestion of raw or undercooked meat containing cysts. During infection in pregnant women, the virulence of the *Trichinella* strain, the trimester of pregnancy in which the infection occurs, and the invasion intensity determine the effect on pregnancy. Patients may have gastroenteritis, then fever, edema, and muscle pain. The presence of loose mucous stools, loss of appetite, nausea, vomiting, and pains in the lower part of the abdomen are uncommon, but they appear more frequently in pregnant patients. Hepatomegaly may also be seen. Additional symptoms are pain in muscle groups, especially ocular muscles; nonitching rash; neuromuscular changes; and cardiovascular manifestations including myocarditis, hypokalemia, and arrhythmias due to hypocalcemia. An allergic reaction early in the disease may cause Loeffler's pneumonia, bronchospasm, and pleural effusions. Later, bacterial superinfection with pneumonia may develop. *Trichinella* larvae may cross the placenta and enter the fetal circulation.

Diagnosis is made by epidemiologic history, clinical signs and symptoms, presence of eosinophilia and leukocytosis, and serology. Elevated creatine kinase and lactate dehydrogenase levels are nonspecific. Serology, beginning in the second week of disease, is most useful with ELISA and passive hemagglutination (PA) tests being the most sensitive. Indirect IFA testing is less sensitive. The PA and ELISA tests remain positive for a few years, but the IFA test usually reverts to negative after one year (12). In the third week of disease, flocculation or agglutination techniques become positive. They have a low sensitivity but high specificity and remain elevated for several years. Muscle biopsy (if positive) is diagnostic. As soon as trichinosis is diagnosed, treatment should be instituted.

Schistosomiasis

Schistosomiasis is caused by blood flukes with the most important species causing human disease being *Schistosoma haematobium* in the Middle East and Africa; *Schistosoma mansoni* in Africa, the Carribean Islands, and South America; and *Schistosoma japonicum* in Asia. Diagnostic laboratory data include eosinophilia, identification of schistome eggs in stool or urine or tissue biopsies. Schistosomiasis may cause anemia, hepatic cirrhosis, obstructive uropathy, and jaundice. Maternal complications can be due to direct disease in the genital tract or chronic disease causing debilitation. Rarely, the placenta may be invaded by schistosoma. Only *S japonicum* has been described in congenital infection; it is generally thought that there are no direct fetal effects of schistosomiasis (13,14).

References

1. Carroll CJ, Hurley R, Stanley VC. Criteria for diagnosis of candida vulvovaginitis in pregnant women. J Obstet Gynaecol Br Cmwlth 1973;80:258–263.
2. Fleury FJ. Adult vaginitis. Clin Obstet Gynecol 1981;24:407–438.
3. Goldacre JJ, Watt B, Loudon N, Miline LJR, London JD, Vessey MP. Vaginal microbial flora in normal young women. Br Med J 1979;1:450–453.
4. Potasman I, Leibovitz Z, Sharf M. Candida sepsis in pregnancy and the postpartum period. Rev Infect Dis 1991;13:146–149.
5. Bille J, Edson RS, Roberts GD. Clinical evaluation of the lysis centrifugation blood culture system for the detection of fungemia and comparison with a

conventional biphasic broth blood culture system. J Clin Microbiol 1984; 19:126–128.

6. Schwartz D, Reef S. *Candida albicans* placentitis and funisitis: early diagnosis of congenital candidemia by histopathologic examination of umbilical cord vessels. Ped Infect Dis J 1990;9:661–665.

7. Kida M, Abramowsky CR, Santoscoy C. Cryptococcosis of the placenta in a woman with acquired immunodeficiency syndrome. Hum Pathol 1989;20: 920–921.

8. Powderly WG. Therapy for cryptococcal meningitis in patients with AIDS. Clin Infect Dis 1992;14:54–59.

9. Lee RV. Parasites in pregnancy: the problems of malaria and toxoplasmosis. Clin J Perinatol 1985;15:351–363.

10. Sweet RL, Gibbs RS. Infectious diseases of the female genital tract. Baltimore: Williams & Wilkins, 1985:227–245.

11. Whiteside M, MacLeod C. The acquired immunodeficiency syndrome. In: MacLeod C, ed. Parasitic infections in pregnancy and the newborn. Oxford: Oxford University Press, 1988:168–169.

12. Kociecka W. Trichinosis. In: MacLeod C, ed. Parasitic infections in pregnancy and the newborn. Oxford: Oxford University Press, 1988:216–220.

13. McNeeley DF, Magu MR. Schistosomiasis. In: MacLeod C, ed. Parasitic infections in pregnancy and the newborn. Oxford: Oxford University Press, 1988:227–251.

14. Tietze PE, Jones JE. Parasites during pregnancy. Prim Care 1991;18:96–97.

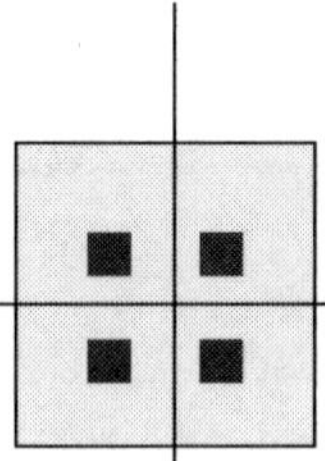

7.
Reproductive Toxicology

Anthony R. Scialli

This chapter addresses the impact of clinical laboratory evaluations in reproductive toxicology. Clinical laboratory testing can be helpful in evaluating exposures that may have an impact on reproductive success. This evaluation may be directed at either of two goals: guiding pharmacologic therapy and identifying the potential for adverse effects on reproduction. The first of these goals presupposes the ability to alter therapy as a result of testing to maximize benefits and minimize the risk of adverse outcome. The second goal is based on the desire to give information to people about damage that may have been done, about possible interventions, or about avoiding future adverse outcomes. These goals are outlined in Table 7-1.

Monitoring Drug Levels

Pharmacologic agents work by achieving an effect at a target site. We give a dose of a drug to get an appropriate number of drug molecules to the target, but rarely are we able to measure how much of the agent gets to the tissue of interest. Instead, we use surrogate measures, particularly concentration of the drug in serum or plasma. Because most drugs are delivered to their targets in blood, it is reasonable to believe that blood levels will reflect tissue levels at equilibrium. In addition, for many drugs, there is substantial experience with correlating blood concentrations and clinical response. Examples of these are listed in Table 7-2.

The physiologic alterations of normal pregnancy may result in changes

TABLE 7-1. Reproduction-related goals of the clinical toxicologist

Scenario	Possible Interventions
I. Guidance of Therapy	
A. Monitoring drug levels	Adjust dose
B. Monitoring toxicity	Adjust dose, change drug, or stop therapy
II. Identifying Potential for Adverse Effects	
A. Finding toxicant present before reproducing	Avoid reproduction until toxicant can be removed
B. Finding toxicant present after conception	Plan diagnostic tests for abnormalities in the conceptus

TABLE 7-2. Examples of clinical correlates with drug concentrations

Drug	Plasma Concentration	Clinical Effect
Phenytoin	10 μg/mL	Seizure control
	20 μg/mL	Nystagmus
	30 μg/mL	Ataxia
	40 μg/mL	Lethargy
Magnesium	8–12 mg/dL	Decreased reflexes
	9–12 mg/dL	Flushing
	10–12 mg/dL	Somnolence, slurred speech
	15–17 mg/dL	Paralysis, respiratory distress
	30–35 mg/dL	Cardiac arrest
Ethanol	20–30 mg/dL	Motor impairment
	100–150 mg/dL	Drunkenness
	400 mg/dL	Respiratory depression

in drug absorption, distribution, biotransformation, and excretion (1). For some agents, the changes in pharmocokinetic parameters make an important difference in whether or not the drug exerts therapeutic effects during pregnancy. Among the best studied in this regard are the anticonvulsants (2). Changes in the handling of these agents are shown in Table 7-3. It should be noted that there is considerable individual response during preg-

TABLE 7-3. Pregnancy-associated changes in pharmacokinetics

Parameter	Alterations
Absorption	Nausea and vomiting may interfere Reduced gastric acid leading to decreased absorption of weak acids and increased absorption of weak bases Decreased gastrointestinal motility with variable effects Increased minute ventilation leading to increased absorption of inhaled agents
Distribution	Decreased plasma albumin leading to altered drug binding Increased plasma volume and total body water Presence of fetal compartment may alter volume of distribution
Biotransformation	Hepatic microsomal enzyme activity may increase
Excretion	Increased glomerular filtration rate Decreased biliary excretion Increased minute ventilation leading to increased pulmonary excretion

nancy, which makes monitoring of plasma concentrations particularly useful in guiding therapy.

In some instances, pregnancy changes are responsible for drug toxicity, even at concentrations not usually considered to be a problem. For example, theophylline is ordinarily about 39% bound to plasma albumin. Because of the decreased albumin concentration in pregnancy, theophylline is about 31% bound in pregnant women (4). Although this represents only a moderate difference in binding, it may result in an increase in unbound drug sufficient to cause symptoms of toxicity at plasma levels ordinarily considered therapeutic. Thus, while a nonpregnant woman may be comfortable at theophylline plasma concentrations of 10–20 μg/mL, during pregnancy, symptoms of theophylline excess may occur if levels exceed 10 μg/mL.

Other laboratory determinations in addition to maternal blood studies may be beneficial. One study evaluating levels of epoxide hydrolase in antenatal evaluation of amniocytes suggests the possibility of antenatal testing for determination of risk for phenytoin embryopathy (3).

Toxicology Screens

The use of body fluids, particularly urine, for the detection of drugs of abuse or their metabolites has become increasingly used in obstetrics. Studies in urban populations of pregnant women have shown alarmingly high rates of positive tests for amphetamines, barbituates, benzodiazepines, cannabinoids, cocaine, phencyclidine, and opioids (5–8). Drug identification can be performed by gas chromatography-mass spectrometry, which is believed to be highly accurate, but screening is generally performed by simple methods such as thin-layer chromatography, enzyme immunoassays, and radioimmunoassays (9). In a blinded evaluation of 31 laboratories across the United States, there were no false positive results and overall accuracy was 97% (10).

Although drugs of abuse have been found in some instances to be human developmental toxicants and although detection of drug abuse by urine screening is possible, there is little evidence that screening programs have altered pregnancy outcome for women at risk. Drug abuse is part of a life-style that may impose pregnancy problems additional to the toxicologic risks. Treatment of pregnant drug-abusing women should address the social and economic issues that contribute to pregnancy outcome (11). To this end, toxicology screens in obstetric populations can be seen as methods to identify women in need, rather than as ends in themselves.

Environmental Agents

The role of environmental pollutants in reproduction has received considerable attention in the lay and scientific press, although data showing effects of these agents are generally restricted to animal studies using high-dose exposures. Among the agents for which there is the greatest concern about human toxicity are heavy metals and cyclic hydrocarbons.

With industrialization has come virtual worldwide contamination of the environment with lead. Although removal of lead from automobile fuels has resulted in decreasing atmospheric lead, the metal persists in soil and is found in storage batteries, paints, and a number of industrial processes. Lead toxicity prominently affects the hematologic and nervous systems. It is currently believed that children with blood lead levels of 25 μg/dL are at risk for intellectual impairment from lead toxicity. Reproductive concerns center around male infertility and miscarriage in addition to central nervous system problems in the developing infant. Although data suggest adverse developmental effects with maternal or cord blood lead concentrations in the range of 10 μg/dL, the methods used to collect these data have been severely criticized (12). In addition, blood lead concentrations may be an imperfect approximation of tissue concentrations or total lead burden.

In managing women with lead exposure, reduction of the exposure before reproduction is advised. If a woman has an elevated blood lead concentration, chelation therapy may be considered. The level at which chelation occurs varies, depending on the attitude toward the controversial data on low-dose effects; however, this "action level" will generally be between 10 and 25 μg/dL.

Polychlorinated biphenyls (PCBs) are associated with developmental effects such as miscarriage, low birthweight, and pigment disorders in the skin and nails (13). Since these agents were banned in 1976, exposure to high levels is unusual; however, some exposure is associated with eating seafood from contaminated waterways. Breast-feeding represents a concern for infants if high PCB exposure is suspected based on history or infant symptoms. The lipid content of milk facilitates excretion of fat-soluble PCBs. Levels of these compounds can be measured in blood or milk. In the presence of high concentrations, breast-feeding might be deferred, but it is unlikely that the benefits of nursing would be outweighed by PCBs in milk except in the most extreme cases.

References

1. Juchau MR, Faustman-Watts E. Pharmacokinetic considerations in the maternal-placental-fetal unit. Clin Obstet Gynecol 1983;26:379–390.
2. Scialli AR. Anticonvulsants in pregnancy. In: Niebyl JR, ed. Drug use in pregnancy. 2d ed. Philadelphia: Lea and Febiger, 1988.
3. Buehler BA, Delimont D, van Waes M, Finnell RH. Prenatal prediction of risk of the fetal hydantoin syndrome. N Engl J Med 1990;322:1567–1572.
4. Connelly TJ, Ruo TI, Frederiksen MC, Atkinson AJ Jr. Characterization of theophylline binding to serum proteins in pregnant and nonpregnant women. Clin Pharmacol Ther 1990;47:68–72.
5. Neerhof MG, MacGregor SN, Retzky SS, Sullivan TP. Cocaine abuse during pregnancy: peripartum prevalence and perinatal outcome. Am J Obstet Gynecol 1989;161:633–638.
6. Matera C, Warren WB, Moomjy M, Fink DJ, Fox HE. Prevalence of use of cocaine and other substances in an obstetric population. Am J Obstet Gynecol 1990;163:797–801.
7. Land DB, Kushner R. Drug abuse during pregnancy in an inner-city hospital: prevalence and patterns. J Am Osteopath Assoc 1990;90:421–426.

8. Osterloh JD, Lee BL. Urine drug screening in mothers and newborns. Am J Dis Child 1989;143:791–793.
9. McCunney RJ. Drug testing: technical complications of a complex social issue. Am J Ind Med 1989;15:589–600.
10. Frings CS, Battaglia DJ, White RM. Status of drugs-of-abuse testing in urine under blind conditions: an AACC study. Clin Chem 1989;35:891–894.
11. Benkendorf JL. Prenatal substance abuse; a ubiquitous cry for help (editorial). Reprod Toxicol 1991;5:87–88.
12. Ernhart C. Critical review of low level prenatal lead exposure in the human. Reprod Toxicol 1992;6:9–19.
13. Lione A. Polychlorinated biphenyls and reproduction. Reprod Toxicol 1988; 2:83–89.

8.
Erythroblastosis Fetalis

John T. Queenan

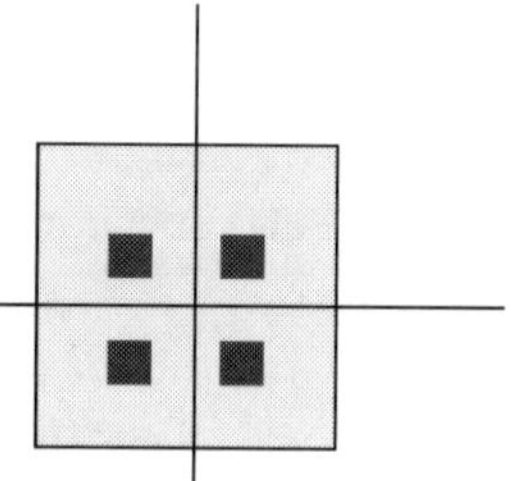

Erythroblastosis fetalis (EBF) poses a wide range of risks to the fetus and the newborn. The Rh-negative mother becomes immunized to the Rh antigen on fetal erythrocytes by means of transplacental hemorrhages (TPH) during the current or prior pregnancy, abortion, or ectopic pregnancy. Rarely, the immunization may be due to an inadvertent transfusion of Rh-positive blood.

The mother develops IgG antibodies, which freely cross the placenta and attack the Rh-positive fetal erythrocytes. Although Rh immunization does not cause symptoms in the mother, the disease in the fetus may range from a mild hemolytic anemia, requiring no therapy, to early fetal death. Clinical laboratory evaluation is crucial in determining risk, detecting isoimmunization, assessing severity of disease in the fetus, and guiding treatment. The goals of testing and the specific laboratory tests used are listed in Table 8-1.

Type and Screen, Antibody Identification, and Titer

On the first prenatal visit, a blood group, Rh type, and antibody screen are performed. The antibody screen is designed to detect Rh antibodies in Rh-negative women and irregular antibodies both in Rh-positive and Rh-negative women. If the antibody screen is positive, the laboratory should identify the antibody and perform a dilution titer to indicate the relative strength of the antibody. In addition to Rh°(D) antigen, other blood group antigens may cause maternal immunizations. A partial list of atypical or irregular antibodies is found in Table 8-2.

TABLE 8-1. Testing for erythroblastosis fetalis

Testing Goals	*Tests Used*
1. Assessing maternal risk, detection of isoimmunization	Blood group and Rh type Antibody screen
2. Paternal testing	Antigen determination
3. Detection of fetal maternal blood	Rosette test Kleihauer-Betke
4. Assessment of disease severity	
A. Maternal testing	Antibody titer
B. Fetal testing	
Amniotic fluid	Amniotic fluid ΔOD_{450}
Cordocentesis	Hemoglobin/hematocrit Blood group/Rh Direct Coombs' Kleihauer-Betke
Sonography	Direct fetal imaging

TABLE 8-2. Atypical or irregular antibodies in erythroblastosis fetalis

Blood Group System	*Antigens Related to Hemolytic Disease*	*Severity of EBF*
Kell	K	Mild to severe
Kidd	Jk^a, Jk^b	Mild to severe
Duffy	Fy^a, Fy^b	Mild to severe
Lutheran	Lu^a, Lu^b	Mild
MNSs	M	Mild to severe
	N	Mild
	S	Mild to severe
	s	Mild to severe
Lewis	Not a proven cause of EBF	No EBF
I	Not a proven cause of EBF	No EBF

In the case of Lewis or I immunizations, the antibodies are almost always large molecule IgM antibodies that do not cross the placenta and, therefore, there is no EBF

Antibody titers are the mainstay of fetal evaluation and are particularly helpful in pregnancies that begin with no antibody present. If a patient's antibody screen is negative on her initial prenatal visit but is found to be 1:8 when evaluating her for Rh immune globulin (RhIG) prophylaxis at 28 weeks, active immunization is identified. If the titer remains low, for example, at 1:8 to 1:16 throughout the remainder of the pregnancy, EBF should be mild. If the titer rises rapidly to 1:128 or 1:256 or greater, it is likely that the fetal hemolysis will be severe (1,2).

If the antibody titer is already significantly elevated at the start of pregnancy, additional antibody studies are of little value because the mother is already fully immunized. For mothers with rising or high titers, amniotic fluid optical density analysis or cordocentesis is necessary to determine the fetal condition and the need for potential therapy.

Erythrocyte Rosette Test

The erythrocyte rosette test provides a rapid laboratory screening test to detect fetal erythrocytes in the maternal circulation (3). This test is qualitative. If erythrocytes are present, then a Kleihauer-Betke test is indicated to quantify the magnitude of the TPH.

Kleihauer-Betke Stain

The Kleihauer-Betke staining detects fetal erythrocytes in the maternal circulation and is extremely valuable when large TPHs are suspected, as can occur in situations of abdominal trauma, spontaneous TPH, external version, or premature separation of the placenta. The number of fetal erythrocytes in relation to the number of adult erythrocytes indicates the size of the TPH. One fetal erythrocyte per 5000 adult erythrocytes is approximately equivalent to a TPH of 1 mL whole blood. A dose of 300 μg RhIG is sufficient to protect against 30 mL of Rh-positive whole blood (4).

Assessing Paternal Antigen Status

If a mother is Rh negative, it is important to know the father's Rh type. If he is Rh negative, no RhIG is necessary.

When an Rh-negative mother becomes Rh immunized, it is valuable to know the Rh zygosity of the father. If she becomes immunized during the course of a pregnancy, it is reasonable to assume that the fetus is Rh positive. When she enters her next pregnancy, it is important to know whether or not the father is homozygous or heterozygous for the Rh factor. If the father is D/D, he is Rh positive, homozygous and all babies will be Rh positive. If he is D/d, he is Rh positive, heterozygous and there is a 50/50 chance of a baby being Rh positive.

Testing for paternal antigen status is advised when the mother has a significant immunization that is possibly not due to the father. For instance, a maternal Kell immunization might be the result of a prior blood transfusion. If the father is Kell negative, there is no need for amniocentesis or cordocentesis to evaluate fetal condition because there will be no hemolytic disease in the fetus.

Amniotic Fluid Analysis

The amniotic fluid deviation in optical density at 450 nm (AF ΔOD_{450}) in an Rh-immunized pregnant patient is an ideal test of fetal condition (5–8). If the clinician fully understands the physiologic properties of amniotic fluid and the pathophysiology of Rh disease, virtually no serious fetal deterioration can be undetected.

Current Method: Recently, Queenan and coworkers presented a method based on an analysis of 789 single and serial AF ΔOD_{450} values in Rh-immunized pregnancies from 14–40 weeks' gestation (9). The advantage of this method is that it is efficacious in both the second and third trimester. In addition, it integrates the complimentary modalities of AF ΔOD_{450} cordocentesis and sonographic monitoring (9).

In normal (Rh-negative fetus) pregnancies, the AF ΔOD_{450} values rise until 24 weeks, then they fall until term. In Rh-positive fetuses at risk of dying in utero, the values are higher and the trends rise. This clinical management scheme consists of four zones of increasing severity (Figure 8-1):

Rh negative (unaffected)
Indeterminate
Rh positive (affected)
Intrauterine death risk

Table 8-3 outlines a clinical management scheme using the four zones. Rh-negative fetuses have minimal invasive procedures. Fetuses at risk of death have early cordocentesis for evaluation and therapy. Values that fall in between can be separated into two zones based on the degree of risk.

If an AF ΔOD_{450} value falls in the intrauterine death risk zone, or if the trend of values will cross over into the zone, the fetus is in jeopardy of dying in utero. Cordocentesis should be performed to determine fetal condition and, when indicated, to provide access for intrauterine transfusions.

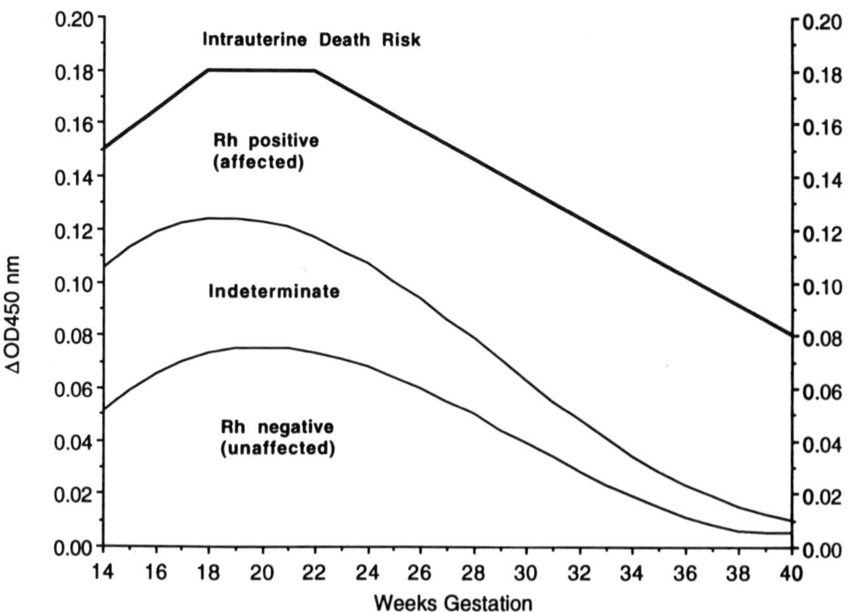

FIGURE 8-1. Four zones of amniotic fluid optical density values are used for detecting fetal condition.

TABLE 8-3. Management

Zone	Action
Intrauterine death risk	Cordocentesis; transfuse as indicated
Rh positive	Repeat amniocentesis q1–2wk; cordocentesis as clinically indicated
Indeterminant	Repeat amniocentesis q2–4wk
Rh negative	Repeat amniocentesis × 1 as clinically indicated; deliver at term

If the value falls in the Rh-negative (unaffected) zone, the fetus can be presumed to be Rh-negative (no EBF). To ensure that the fetus is unaffected, an additional amniocentesis may be necessary.

If the AF ΔOD_{450} value falls in either of the middle zones, subsequent amniotic fluid values are necessary to indicate the condition of the fetus.

TABLE 8-4. Normal fetal hemoglobin and hematocrit values

Weeks of Gestation	Hematocrit (%)	Hemoglobin (g/dL)
18–20	35.8	11.4
21–22	38.5	12.2
23–25	38.6	12.4
26–30	41.5	13.3

Decreasing values generally mean that the fetus is Rh positive with mild or moderate EBF or even Rh negative (unaffected). Rising trends indicate severe disease. Horizontal trends can be associated with severe disease and even death if the fetus is not delivered or transfused depending on gestational age.

Cordocentesis

Cordocentesis is indicated to detect a life-threatening hemolytic anemia in the fetus and provide access for intravascular transfusion at the same time (1). A fetal hematocrit is performed immediately. If significant fetal anemia is detected, an intravascular transfusion is done. Forestier and colleagues have determined normal values for fetal hematocrits and hemoglobins according to weeks of gestation (Table 8-4; 10). The blood is also submitted for a blood group Rh and direct Coombs' test, and Kleihauer-Betke stain to confirm fetal origin.

Sonography

Direct imaging of the fetus is an excellent complement to laboratory testing. If the fetus deteriorates due to the hemolytic anemia, certain sonographic characteristics will be evident (1). Pericardial effusion and cardiomegaly are early signs. Fetal ascites and polyhydramnios are also good indicators of fetal deterioration. Hydropic changes in the fetus are almost always present when the fetal hematocrit drops to the 15% area.

References

1. Queenan JT. Rh and other blood group immunizations. In: Queenan JT, ed. Management of high risk pregnancy, 3d ed. Boston: Blackwell Scientific Publications, 1994:423.
2. Queenan JT. Modern management of the Rh problem, 2d ed. Baltimore: Harper & Row, 1977:33.

3. Stedman CM, Baudin JC, White CA, Cooper ES. Use of the erythrocyte rosette test to screen for excessive fetomaternal hemorrhage in Rh-negative women. Am J. Obstet Gynecol 1986;154:1363–1369.
4. Kleihauer E, Braun H, Betke K. Demonstration von fetalem Hamoglobin in den Erythrocyten ein Blutasstichs. Klin Wochenschr 1957;35:637.
5. Liley AW. Liquor amnii analysis in management of pregnancy complicated by Rhesus sensitization. Am J Obstet Gynecol 1961;82:1359–1370.
6. Liley AW. Errors in the assessment of haemolytic disease from amniotic fluid. Am J Obstet Gynecol 1963;86:485–494.
7. Queenan JT, Goetschel E. Amniotic fluid analysis for erythroblastosis fetalis. Obstet Gynecol 1968;32:120–133.
8. Whitfield CR. A three-year assessment of an action line method of timing intervention in Rhesus isoimmunization. Am J Obstet Gynecol 1970;108:1239–1244.
9. Queenan JT, Tomai TP, Ural SH, King JC. Deviation in amniotic fluid optical density at a wavelength of 450 nm in Rh-immunized pregnancies from 14–40 weeks' gestation: a proposal for clinical management. Am J Obstet Gynecol 1993;168:1370–1376.
10. Forestier F, Daffos F, Galacteros F, et al. Hematological values of 163 normal fetuses between 18 and 30 weeks of gestation. Pediatr Res 1986;20:342–346.

9.
Nonimmune Hydrops

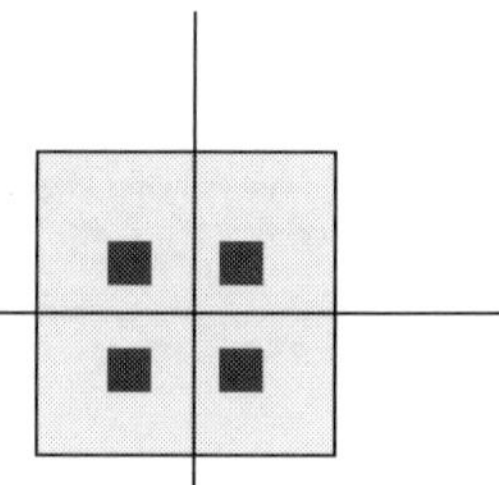

Shaun G. Lencki

Hydrops fetalis was first recognized 100 years ago by Ballantyne. The term hydrops refers to the abnormal accumulation of fluid in one or more serous cavities of the fetus. Hydrops can be divided into two groups—immune and nonimmune. Additional information regarding immune hydrops can be found in Chapter 8. The incidence of nonimmune hydrops is 1 in 2500-3500 pregnancies (1) and is now more common than immune hydrops. The perinatal mortality rate ranges from 50% to 98% and is highly dependent upon the cause (2). Table 9-1 lists the major categories and principle etiologies. Cardiovascular and idiopathic causes make up a large number of the cases of nonimmune hydrops (3,4). Sonography and echocardiography play important roles in the diagnosis of cardiac, renal, gastrointestinal, and placental etiologies for hydrops. This chapter focuses on clinical laboratory evaluation of nonimmune hydrops and primarily discusses laboratory testing for hematologic, chromosomal, and infectious etiologies. Table 9-2 presents an overview of this testing beginning with the separation of immune from nonimmune hydrops using the indirect Coombs' test.

Hematologic Studies

The principle entities of concern under this category include severe maternal anemia, fetal α-thalassemia, glucose-6-phosphate dehydrogenase (G6PD) deficiency, and Gaucher's disease. A complete blood count will establish the presence of maternal anemia. If a microcytic anemia is

TABLE 9-1. Conditions associated with nonimmune hydrops

Cardiovascular

Rhythm disorders
Anatomic defects
Cardiomyopathy
Myocarditis (Coxsackie virus or CMV)

Chromosomal

Trisomy 13, 18, and 21
Turner syndrome
XX/XY mosaicism
Triploidy

Malformation syndromes

A large number have been noted including:
 Thanatophoric dwarfism
 Arthrogryposis multiplex congenita
 Achondroplasia
 Osteogenesis imperfecta

Twin pregnancy

Twin-twin transfusion syndrome

Hematologic

α-Thalassemia
G6PD deficiency
Gaucher's disease
(secondary to marrow infiltration)

Urinary

Urethral stenosis
Urethral valves
Congenital nephrosis (Finnish type)
Prune belly syndrome
Renal dysplasia
Wilms' tumor

Respiratory

Diaphragmatic hernia
Pulmonary sequestration
Pulmonary hypoplasia

Gastrointestinal

Jejunal atresia
Midgut volvulus
Intestinal malrotation
Intestinal duplication
Meconium peritonitis

Liver

Hepatic fibrosis
Cholestasis
Biliary atresia
Familial cirrhosis

Maternal

Severe diabetes mellitus
Severe anemia
Hypoproteinemia
Toxemia

Placental/umbilical cord

Chorangioma
Fetomaternal transfusion
Thrombotic complication
Umbilical cord torsion or
true knot

Medications

Indomethacin
(fetal ductus closure)

TABLE 9-1, continued

Infections	Congenital hepatitis
	Herpes simplex
CMV	Rubella
Parvovirus	Leptospirosis
Coxsackie B	Chagas' disease
Toxoplasmosis	
Syphilis	

TABLE 9-2. Laboratory diagnosis of nonimmune hydrops

Indirect Coombs' Test

Positive: Immune Hydrops	*Negative: Nonimmune Hydrops*
Serial antibody screens	*Other studies*
Amniocentesis for ΔOD_{450}	Genetic history/pedigree
Cordocentesis when indicated	Level II ultrasound
	Fetal echocardiogram

Lab evaluation

Maternal studies	Fetal studies
CBC	Karyotype
If microcytic anemia	Amniotic fluid
then ferritin, hemoglobin electrophoresis	CMV culture
If macrocytic then folate/B_{12}	Enzyme assay
Glucose (diabetic eval)	Gaucher's etc
VDRL/rapid plasma reagin	Cordocentesis
Kleihauer-Betke stain	Hematocrit/hemoglobin
Titers for:	Protein level
Toxoplasmosis	Viral IgM titers
CMV	DNA probe assay
Parvovirus	Hemoglobin electrophoresis
Coxsackie B	

present (mean corpuscular volume [MCV] < 80 fl), serum iron and total iron binding capacity should be assayed to exclude iron deficiency anemia. In the absence of iron deficiency anemia, a hemoglobin electrophoresis should be performed. A normal hemoglobin electrophoresis in this situation may suggest α-thalassemia as the etiology for the hydrops.

Parental serum DNA analysis is required to confirm the heterozygote carrier status. The hydropic fetus with α-thalassemia will have > 80% hemoglobin Bart's (5) detectable on cordocentesis.

If the maternal MCV is normal, then other causes of anemia should be investigated such as hemolytic anemia and anemia of chronic disease. A macrocytic anemia (MCV > 100 fl) may represent a folate or vitamin B_{12} deficiency.

Nonimmune hydrops has been associated with G6PD deficiency. The overabundance of oxidants (nicotinamide-adenine dinucleo-tide) leads to red cell hemolysis. Because it is transmitted as an X-linked disorder, it is most evident in males. The heterozygotic female, however, may exhibit milder symptoms if the normal X chromosome is inactivated (Lyon's hypothesis). Maternal screening should rely on quantitated enzyme analysis and not qualitative dye studies (6).

In the rarely occurring Gaucher's disease, the fetal bone marrow can be extensively infiltrated with Gaucher's cells. This can lead to severe anemia and hydrops. Prenatal diagnosis is available through amniocyte culture and measurement of glucocerebrosidase activity.

Chromosomal Analysis

Chromosomal aneuploidy, such as monosomy X (Turner syndrome), trisomy 21 (Down syndrome), trisomy 18 (Edward syndrome), and trisomy 13 (Patau syndrome) has been associated with nonimmune hydrops. Turner syndrome accounted for the majority of cases of nonimmune hydrops before 21 weeks' gestation in a series of 30 pregnancies (7).

Decisions regarding chorionic villous sampling, amniocentesis, or cordocentesis depend on time of the diagnosis, urgency of obtaining results, prior history of hydrops, and wishes of the parents. Karyotypes from fetal white cells obtained at the time of cordocentesis may be available in 3 days. In cases of hydrops associated with oligohydramnios, chorionic villous sampling may be helpful when amniocentesis is prohibited.

Kleihauer-Betke Stain

The possibility of a chronic maternal-fetal hemorrhage must not be overlooked. The Kleihauer-Betke stain is an acid elution assay that denatures adult hemoglobin in the red blood cells. Fetal hemoglobin is not affected and remains stable. The fetal cells in the maternal circulation can be quantitated in milliliters by most hematology laboratories. Case reports by Rouse and Weiner (8) and Tannirandorn and colleagues (9) demonstrated volumes of 230 mL and 113 mL, respectively, in the maternal circulation in cases of nonimmune hydrops.

Infectious Disease Evaluation

There is a strong association between syphilis and nonimmune hydrops. The fetus and the placenta infected by *Treponema pallidum* become edematous. The fluorescent treponemal antibody absorption test or microhemagglutination test should also be performed. Recently, Berkowitz and coworkers reported data on 4 cases of nonimmune hydrops with false negative nonspecific antibody tests (10). The authors raise the issue of suboptimal flocculation due to a prozone effect with nontreponemal assays. The prozone effect may be avoided if serial dilution of serum samples for rapid plasma reagin or VDRL is performed prior to the assay.

Serology is equally important in the diagnosis of cytomegalovirus (CMV) as in syphilis. The presence of serum IgG in the maternal blood does not necessarily confer complete protection. Recurrent CMV infection during pregnancy represents a risk to the fetus even in the presence of CMV-specific IgG. The fetal risk from a recurrent infection is much lower ($< 5\%$) than a primary infection in pregnancy (30% to 50%; 11). Fetal exposure may be clarified by amniotic fluid CMV culture and cordocentesis for nonspecific total IgM titers and γ-glutamyl transferase (12).

Studies for toxoplasmosis use the Sabin-Feldman assay at most reference laboratories. This assay is performed with methylene blue dye. The dilutional titer at which half the parasites are stained and half are unstained is reported (13). Either seroconversion or a fourfold increase in serial IgG toxospecific titers drawn 3-4 weeks apart represents an acute infection. Other tests of recent infection are the IgM fluorescent antibody assay and the IgM enzyme-linked immunosorbent assay. To determine fetal exposure, cordocentesis may be performed for IgM-specific antibodies using these assays. The most reliable test remains the peritoneal animal culture; unfortunately, this may take up to 6 weeks for results. Holliman and colleagues published a case report to illustrate the difficulty of antenatal diagnosis of congenital toxoplasmosis by serologic and DNA probe techniques (14). Maternal contamination of serologic assays can lead to false positive results.

Additional testing for an infectious etiology for nonimmune hydrops includes evaluation for parvovirus (15-17) and coxsackie B virus (18). This will be discussed in further detail in Part 7. For patients from South and

Central America, Chagas' disease should be considered. Maternal infection may lead to fetal cardiomyopathy and hydrops. Laboratory diagnosis depends on cultures, isolation on peripheral smears, and serology.

References

1. Holzgreve W, Curry C, Golbus M, Callen P, Filly R, Smith JC. Investigation of nonimmune hydrops fetalis. Am J Obstet Gynecol 1984;150:805–812.
2. Castillo RA, DeVoe LD, Hadi HA, Martin S, Geist D. Nonimmune hydrops fetalis: clinical experience and factors related to poor outcome. Am J Obstet Gynecol 1986;155:812–816.
3. Poeschmann RP, Verheijen RH, Van Dongen PW. Differential diagnosis and causes of nonimmunological hydrops fetalis: a review. Obstet Gynecol Surv 1991;46:223–231.
4. Warsof SL, Nicolaides KH, Rodeck C. Immune and non-immune hydrops. Clin Obstet Gynecol 1986;29:533–542.
5. Nakayama R, Yamada D, Steinmiller V, Hsia E, Hale R. Hydrops fetalis secondary to Bart's hemoglobinopathy. Obstet Gynecol 1986;67:176–180.
6. Henry JB. Clinical diagnosis and management by laboratory methods, 17th ed. Philadelphia: WB Saunders, 1984:688–689.
7. Brown BS. The ultrasonographic features of nonimmune hydrops fetalis: a study of 30 successive patients. Can Assoc Radiol J 1986;37:164–168.
8. Rouse D, Weiner C. Ongoing fetomaternal hemorrhage treated by fetal intravascular transfusion. Obstet Gynecol 1990;76:974–975.
9. Tannirandorn Y, Nicolini U, Nicolaidis P, Nasrat H, Letsky EA, Rodeck CH. Intrauterine death due to fetomaternal hemorrhage despite successful treatment of fetal anemia. J Perinat Med 1990;18:233–235.
10. Berkowitz K, Baxi L, Fox HE. False-negative syphilis screening: the prozone phenomenon, nonimmune hydrops, and diagnosis of syphilis during pregnancy. Am J Obstet Gynecol 1990;163:975–977.
11. Gilbert GL. Congenital and perinatal cytomegalovirus infections. Aust N Z Obstet Gynecol 1985:25:169–172.
12. Lynch L, Daffos R, Emanuel D, Giovangrandi Y, Meisel R, Forestier F. Prenatal diagnosis of fetal cytomegalovirus infection. Am J Obstet Gynecol 1991; 156:714–718.
13. Remington J, Klein J. Infectious disease of the fetus and newborn infant, 3d ed. Philadelphia: WB Saunders, 1990:154–158.
14. Holliman RE, Johnson JD, Constantine G, Bissenden JG, Nicolaides K, Savva D. Difficulties in the diagnosis of congenital toxoplasmosis by cordocentesis. Case report. Br J Obstet Gynaecol 1991;98:832–834.
15. Anderson LJ, Hurwitz ES. Human parvovirus B19 and pregnancy. Clin Perinatol 1988;15:273–286.

16. Anand A, Gray ES, Brown T, Clewley JP, Cohen BJ. Human parvovirus infection in pregnancy and hydrops fetalis. N Engl J Med 1987;316:183–186.

17. Peters MT, Nicolaides KH. Cordocentesis for the diagnosis and treatment of human fetal parvovirus infection. Obstet Gynecol 1990;75:501–504.

18. Rotbart HA. Nucleic acid detection systems for enteroviruses. Clin Microbiol Rev 1991;4:156–168.

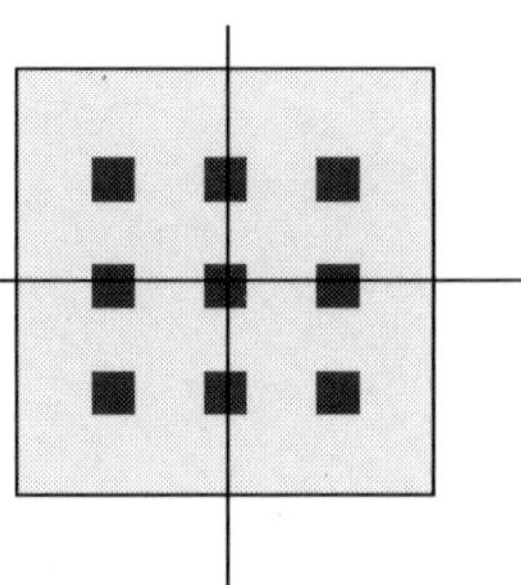

PART THREE
Genetics

10.

Genetic Laboratory Diagnosis

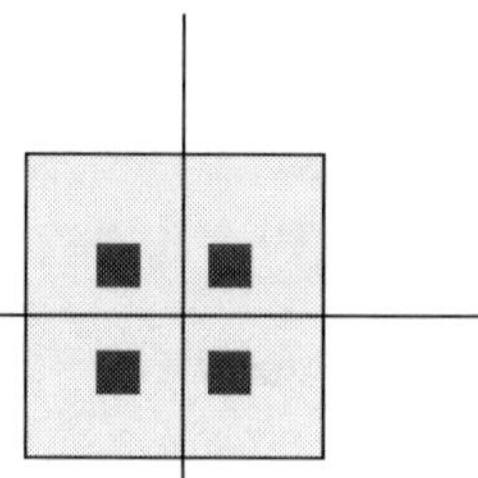

Thomas L. Pinckert

The prenatal diagnosis of congenital anomalies is a topic of great importance to practitioners and parents alike. Although the merits of each test used in prenatal diagnosis must be weighed in terms of its risk/benefit ratio, any test that helps confirm fetal well-being is generally readily accepted. A broad overview of prenatal laboratory testing used in genetic diagnosis is presented.

Cytogenetics

Table 10-1 presents the indications for cytogenetic testing (karyotyping). Testing can be performed on a number of different tissue types that include leukocytes (parental and fetal cordocentesis), trophoblasts (chorionic villus sampling, aborted material), amniocytes (amniocentesis), and fetal skin or muscle. Cytogenetic testing can identify aneuploidy, structural chromosome abnormalities, and mosaicism.

Triple Screen

Evaluation of α-fetoprotein (AFP), unconjugated estriol (uE3), and human chorionic gonadotropin (hCG) are presently being used at 15–20 weeks' gestation to ascertain risks for Down syndrome. This testing allows for screening of younger women who do not have the age-related risk found in women 35 and older. Low levels of AFP and uE3 and elevated levels of hCG are associated with an increased risk of Down syndrome. Second trimester risk levels $\geq$ 1:190 have been suggested as the level at

---

TABLE 10-1. **Indications for cytogenetic testing**

Maternal age
History of aneuploidy in prior pregnancy
Sonographic demonstration of fetal abnormality/
  hydrops
Risk indication by triple screening
Habitual abortion
Balanced parental chromosome rearrangement

---

which to offer amniocentesis for chromosome analysis. Use of the triple screen in women over age 35 has been investigated, but it should be remembered that this form of testing does not in itself diagnose or rule out Down syndrome. Recent studies have shown a correlation of trisomy 18 with decreased levels of AFP, uE3, and hCG. Triple screen studies have not shown risk prediction for trisomy 13.

Enzymes Studies

An example of this testing is the measurement of hexosaminidase A activity in carrier identification and prenatal diagnosis of Tay-Sachs disease. In carrier identification, serum levels are used except in pregnant women or those taking oral contraceptives. Leukocyte assays take the place of serum determinations in those settings. DNA testing has also been developed for Tay-Sachs screening and complements the enzyme analyses. Several biochemical tests have been developed to aid the clinician in the prenatal diagnosis of rare metabolic diseases. The reader is referred to more comprehensive texts for a complete discussion.

Laboratory Testing for Neural Tube Defects

α-Fetoprotein and acetylcholinesterase (AChE) are the primary laboratory tests used in prenatal diagnosis of neural tube defects. Table 10-2 lists the conditions associated with elevated levels of these two substances. Present screening protocols assess maternal serum AFP drawn at 15–20 weeks' gestation. Laboratory values are adjusted for maternal weight, race, and insulin-dependent diabetes. Levels in the range of 2.0–2.5 multiples of the median (MOM) necessitate repeat studies and sonography. If repeat AFP is elevated and sonography indicates that the gestational dates have not been miscalculated, then high-resolution sonography and amnio-

TABLE 10-2. Conditions associated with elevations in α-fetoprotein and acetylcholinesterase

Elevated Maternal Serum AFP	Elevated Amniotic Fluid AFP	Positive AChE
Incorrect dates	Fetal blood	Strong specific band
Multiple gestation	contamination	Neural tube defect
Fetal anomalies	Fetal anomalies	some cases of:
Neural tube defects	Neural tube defects	Cystic hygroma
Ventral wall defects	Ventral wall defects	Broad nondistinct fast
Gastrointestinal	Gastrointestinal	band
obstruction	obstruction	Blood
Renal nephrosis	Renal nephrosis	contamination
Teratoma	Teratoma	Broad, nonspecific
Cystic hygroma	Cystic hygroma	band and weak spe-
Placental abnormality	Placental abnormality	cific band
Amniotic bands	Amniotic bands	Ventral wall defect
Chorangioma	Chorangioma	
Villitis	Villitis	
Infections	Infections	
Cytomegalovirus	Cytomegalovirus	
Parvovirus	Parvovirus	
Hepatitis	Hepatitis	
Fetomaternal bleeding		
Maternal malignancy		
Hepatocellular		
carcinoma		
Yolk sac tumor		

centesis are recommended. If the amniotic fluid AFP level is $> 2.0–2.5$ MOM, AChE electrophoretic determinations are also performed. The band pattern analysis of AChE helps not only to complement the AFP in risk assessment but also helps to assess for false elevations of AFP due to fetal blood contamination.

In approximately 30% of patients with an elevated maternal serum AFP no etiology can be determined even after a targeted level II ultrasound, amniocentesis, and normal biochemical marker analysis. These patients have been extensively studied and should be considered as high risk. In-creased incidences of premature delivery, low birthweight, placental abruption, fetal demise, and later development of preeclampsia have been identified in these patients.

Fetal Blood Studies

Fetal blood sampling or cordocentesis procedures for genetic diagnosis may be indicated when prior genetic testing has been unsuccessful, in late registrants with risk factors, or when sonography has identified fetal anomalies or nonimmune hydrops. Rapid karyotyping, hemoglobin studies, biochemical evaluations, and DNA-based testing are possible to aid the clinician in prenatal diagnosis.

Molecular Diagnostics

Prenatal diagnosis through molecular diagnostic techniques has grown exponentially due to identification of gene mutations and general advances in molecular technology (restriction enzymes, cloning, blotting, amplification by polymerase chain reaction) α_1-Antitrypsin deficiency, Duchenne muscular dystrophy, fragile X syndrome, Gaucher's disease, Tay-Sachs disease, hemophilia, sickle cell anemia, thalassemia, and von Willebrand's disease represent just a small component of diseases in which DNA-based diagnostic tests play a role. Molecular techniques show applicability in diseases where the molecular basis is not known through use of restriction fragment length polymorphisms that have been evaluated in affected family members.

Significant advances have been made recently in DNA-based carrier testing and prenatal diagnosis of cystic fibrosis (CF). Carrier screening is recommended when an individual has an affected family member. Although many CF mutations have been described in addition to $\Delta508$, approximately 88% of Caucasian CF carriers are determined when testing is performed on up to 22 of the more common mutations.

In fluorescent in situ hybridization (FISH), the laboratory uses DNA probes that bind to homologous sequences in metaphase chromosomes or interphase nuclei (thus eliminating the need for culture). Probes can vary from smaller unique sequence probes to whole chromosome probes. Probes are presently available that allow for identification of aneuploidy (13,18,21,X,Y). It is hoped that future applications of this method will allow for aneuploidy screening of fetal cells that have been obtained from maternal blood.

Suggested Reading

Brock DJH, Sutcliffe RG. Alpha fetoprotein in the antenatal diagnosis of anencephaly and spina bifida. Lancet 1972;2:197–199.

Haddow JE. Prenatal screening for open neural tube defects, Down's syndrome, and other major fetal disorders. Semin Perinatol 1990;14:488–503.

Haddow JE, Palomaki GE, Knight GJ, et al. Prenatal screening for Down's syndrome with use of maternal serum markers. N Engl J Med 1992;327:588–593.

King CR. Genetic linkage: the basis of human gene mapping. Obstet Gynecol Surv 1989;44:177–189.

King CR. Prenatal diagnosis of genetic disease with molecular genetic technology. Obstet Gynecol Surv 1988;43:493–508.

Merkatz IR, Nitowsky HM, Macri JN, Johnson WE. An association between low maternal serum alpha-fetoprotein and fetal chromosomal abnormalities. Am J Obstet Gynecol 1984;148:886–891.

Steele MW, Breg WR. Chromosome analysis of human amniotic fluid cells. Lancet 1966;1:383–385.

Wald NJ, Cuckle HS, Densem JW, et al. Maternal serum screening for Down's syndrome in early pregnancy. Br Med J 1988;297:883–887.

11.
Genetic Analysis of
Pregnancy Loss

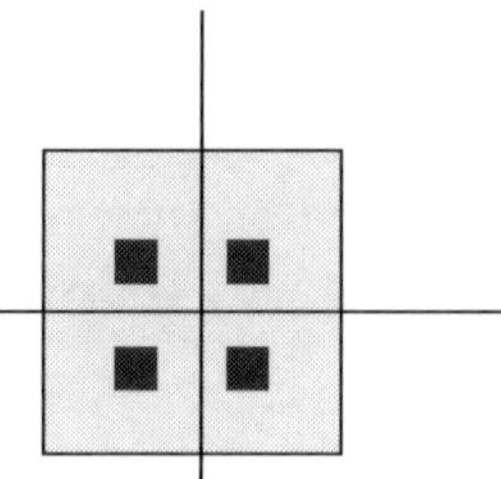

Karin J. Blakemore
Kathryn D. McGowan

Approximately 15% to 20% of clinically recognized pregnancies end in spontaneous loss. The loss of very early embryos, or preembryos, occurs even more frequently. Chromosomal abnormalities play a significant role in this loss. It has now been well established that the rate of chromosomal abnormalities in first trimester abortions is between 50% and 60% (1-5).

The percentage distribution of chromosome abnormalities in spontaneous abortuses is presented in Table 11-1. The most frequent *single chromosomal* abnormality encountered in first trimester abortuses is monosomy X, the cause of Turner syndrome. This represents approximately 18% of the chromosomal anomalies seen. The largest *category* of chromosomal abnormalities found in spontaneous abortions is the autosomal trisomies, which comprise about half of all the chromosome abnormalities seen. The spectrum of trisomies seen in early abortuses, however, is far different from that later in gestation and in live births. Unlike the trisomies seen in live individuals, primarily affecting chromosomes 21, 18, 13, and also the sex chromosomes, early abortuses have been described with every autosomal trisomy except for trisomy for chromosome 1. The most common autosomal trisomy among abortuses involves chromosome 16, which alone accounts for approximately 16% of the total. In contrast, trisomy 16 is not seen in live infants.

Polyploidy represents 20% to 25% of the chromosomal abnormalities found in spontaneous abortions, most commonly triploidy. Although most of these conceptions result in early empty sacs or simply very early

TABLE 11-1. Distribution of chromosome abnormalities in spontaneous abortuses

Trisomies (trisomy 16—16%)	52%
45,X	18%
Triploidy	17%
Tetraploidy	6%
Structural abnormality	3%

miscarriages, some triploid conceptuses survive later into gestation, so-called partial molar pregnancies. This term arose from the edematous changes frequently seen in the placentas of triploid conceptuses, which were reminiscent of complete hydatidiform moles in their gross appearance (6-8). Very few triploid fetuses reach viability, and those that do display characteristic major congenital anomalies.

Structural abnormalities of chromosomes include translocations, inversions, duplications, and deletions. Structural cytogenetic abnormalities comprise < 5% of chromosomally abnormal abortuses. Their presence, however, warrants examination of parental karyotypes. The majority of structural abnormalities occur de novo. Occasionally, however, one parent is found to have a balanced rearrangement of chromosomal material. Although that individual is phenotypically normal, some of his or her gametes will have an unbalanced amount of chromosomal material that can result in an abnormal embryo. This, in turn, can lead to miscarriage. Such couples may come to medical attention from habitual pregnancy losses, or with a positive family history for multiple miscarriages, neonatal deaths, or stillbirths.

Mosaicism has been reported in up to 5% of cytogenetically abnormal spontaneous abortions. Mosaicism refers to the presence of two or more cytogenetically different cell lines in the same specimen or individual. For instance, there may be a normal (46,XX or 46,XY) cell line and a second abnormal cell line. Since the advent of chorionic villus sampling, mosaicism has come to be recognized as a relatively frequent event in many placentas of continuing pregnancies. Mosaicism confined to the placenta is seen in 1% to 2% of chorionic villus samples from viable pregnancies. Although the villi of the early placenta, or chorion frondosum, generally reflect the genotype of the fetus, we now recognize a propensity for placental tissue to exhibit chromosomal mosaicism not actually present in the fetus per se.

Obtaining Samples for Cytogenetic Analysis on Products of Conception

It is relatively simple to obtain adequate tissue samples when cytogenetic study is desired on the products of conception. Chorionic villi can be dissected clean of contaminating maternal decidua so that a reliable fetal karyotype, representative of the conceptus rather than the mother, can be obtained. It is important to obtain tissue samples using sterile technique whenever possible. In most cytogenetic laboratories, long-term cultures are established from the tissue samples submitted, which may take several weeks to grow before the cells are finally harvested. Bacterial or fungal contamination is the most common cause of culture failure in the laboratory. If the tissue sample is unavoidably contaminated, growth may still be successful because the laboratory can initially soak the specimen in a solution containing a high concentration of antibacterial and antifungal agents. "Direct" metaphase preparations involving extremely short culture times will also lessen the risk of bacterial or fungal contamination. These "direct" preparations often yield less than ideal chromosome morphology, but they are generally adequate for counting chromosome number and establishing fetal sex (Figure 11-1).

When cytogenetic analysis is desired at the time of curettage, it is worthwhile requesting if the operating room will supply a sterile bottle or sterile "sock" into which the products of conception will be collected. In addition, the cytogenetics laboratory in your area might be willing to supply a stock of sterile wide-mouth specimen bottles containing minimal essential media that can be stored refrigerated for at least a month, and probably longer. In the absence of any available tissue culture media, the patient's specimen can be sent covered by a piece of sterile gauze that is moistened with normal saline or lactated Ringer's solution. Sterile water should not be used. Neither should the specimen be immersed in normal saline. This may retard the growth in culture. Hank's balanced salt solution is a useful substitute for tissue culture media, and some laboratories have routinely received samples immersed in this, or even in serum from the patient.

Recognizing chorionic villi is relatively easy if one flotates the tissue (Figure 11-2). Chorionic villi, or placental tissue, characteristically fans out into multiple fronds. Maternal decidua tissue generally remains as a

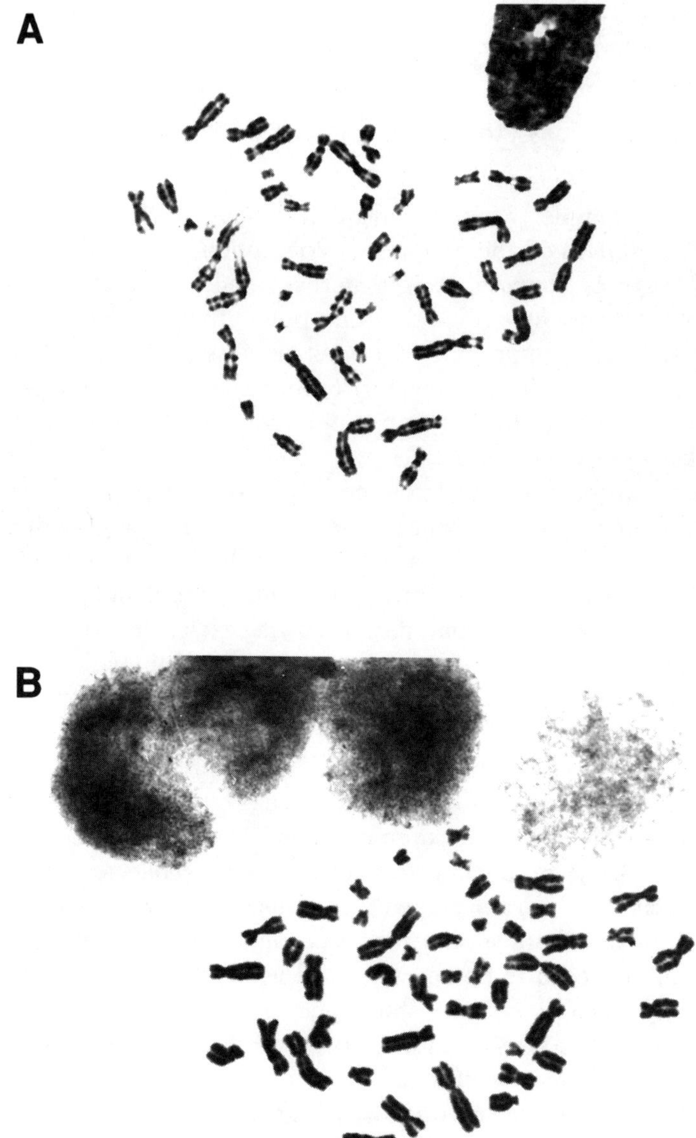

FIGURE 11-1. Stained metaphase preparations: (A) after long-term chorionic villus culture; (B) a "direct" prep after overnight incubation. Better chromosome morphology is apparent in (A) as compared with (B).

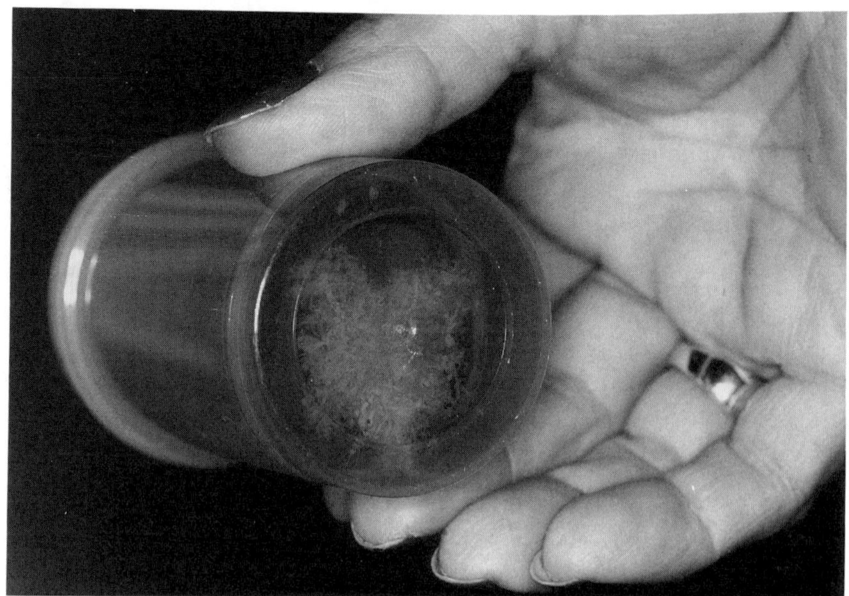

FIGURE 11-2. Chorionic villi, or placental tissue, may be the only viable specimen source for cytogenetic analysis of a spontaneous abortion. Flotation of the specimen in tissue culture media demonstrates the delicate frondlike structure characteristic of chorionic villi.

solid clump. Rinsing the tissue free of blood, using media preferably, can facilitate visualization. It is best not to combine multiple specimens (placenta, fetal skin, etc) to prevent bacterial or fungal cross-contamination. It is less of a problem to recognize placental tissue versus decidua later in gestation and flotation becomes unnecessary. Obtaining a sterile sample following vaginal delivery is the major problem. Expeditious transfer to the laboratory is best, so that antibiotic soaks can be initiated. For fetal skin biopsies, wipe off the area with alcohol several times and use sterile instruments to remove the specimen.

When in utero fetal demise is encountered, the obstetrician may want to consider an amniocentesis if a cytogenetic analysis is desired. There is a high success rate in achieving a cytogenetic diagnosis from amniotic fluid cells, which retain some viability even weeks after fetal demise. In addition, amniotic fluid samples are obtained under sterile conditions. Although it may seem like "bad timing" for a clinician to suggest an amniocentesis to an already distressed patient, the information may ultimately be of great value to her. This procedure or alternatively transabdominal chorionic villus sampling should especially be considered if a chromosomal abnormality is suspected by sonographic detection of fetal anomalies, hydrops, or polyhydramnios.

References

1. Boue J, Boue A, Lazar P. Retrospective and prospective epidemiologic studies of 1500 karyotyped spontaneous human abortions. Teratology 1975;12:11–26.
2. Creasy MR, Crolla JA, Alberman ED. A cytogenetic study of human spontaneous abortions using banding techniques. Hum Genet 1976;31:177–196.
3. Byrne J, Warburton D, Kline J, et al. Morphology of early fetal deaths and their chromosomal characteristics. Teratology 1985;32:297–315.
4. Hassold T, Chen N, Funkhouser J, et al. A cytogenetic study of 1000 spontaneous abortions. Ann Hum Genet 1980;44:151–178.
5. Alberman ED, Creasy MR. Frequency of chromosome abnormalities in miscarriages and perinatal deaths. J Med Genet 1977;14:313–315.
6. Vassilakas P, Riotton G, Kajii H. Hydatidiform mole, two entities: a morphological and cytogenetic study with some clinical considerations. Am J Obstet Gynecol 1977;127:167–170.
7. Szulman AE, Surti U. The syndromes of hydatidiform mole, I: cytogenetic and morphologic correlations. Am J Obstet Gynecol 1978;131:665–671.
8. Szulman AE, Surti U. The syndrome of hydatidiform mole, II: morphologic evolution of the complete and partial mole. Am J Obstet Gynecol 1978; 132:20–27.

12.
Ambiguous Genitalia

Gail F. Whitman

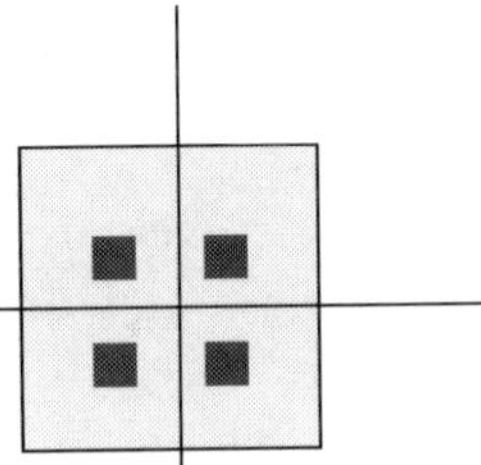

Genital ambiguity discovered in the delivery room presents a medical emergency. Although one may elect to refer these cases to a tertiary care center for evaluation, two life-threatening conditions should be anticipated immediately: salt-wasting congenital adrenal hyperplasia noted in many virilized female infants and congenital hypopituitarism noted in some undermasculinized newborn males. In all cases, every attempt should be made to assign the sex of rearing within the first 48 hours of life.

Immediate Steps

- Review clinical history
- Newborn physical examination
- 17-Hydroxyprogesterone
- Serum electrolytes
- Glucose
- Newborn karyotype
- Maternal androgen levels

17-Hydroxyprogesterone

Until recently the most common cause of female virilization in utero was secondary to maternal androgen ingestion. Today congenital adrenal hyperplasia (CAH) resulting from 21-hydroxylase deficiency is the leading cause. CAH is an autosomal recessive disorder occuring in about 1:5000 to 1:15,000 live births. A markedly elevated serum 17-hydroxyprogesterone level (formerly urinary pregnanetriol) is the primary diagnostic laboratory test. These levels are slightly elevated in all normal newborns for the first 2–3 days of life at which time the levels decline. Thus, at risk infants should be followed closely for several days. The absence of a palpable gonad on newborn physical examination suggests CAH until proven otherwise.

Serum Electrolytes

Fifty percent of the infants with CAH will have significant salt wasting. However, because of the influence of maternal peripartum steroids, many affected newborns will maintain normal electrolyte levels for several days. Electrolytes should be followed for at least 10 days. 21-hydroxylase-deficient salt wasters will have hyponatremia and hyperkalemia.

Glucose

Hypoglycemia in a newborn with micropenis is pathognomonic of congenital hypopituitarism. This is a rare but serious and immediate life threat. Because the small but normally formed penis can be associated with cryptorchidism, these undermasculinized infants may be confused with virilized females. In normal newborns, serum prolactin levels are elevated tenfold over adult levels. This elevation is sustained over the first 4 weeks of life. Infants with hypopituitarism maintain extremely low prolactin levels. This unequivocal finding should aid in a rapid diagnosis.

Karyotype

Determination of gonadal sex is a major component of the evaluation. Because an intra-abdominal gonad with Y chromosome material is prone to malignant degeneration, all newborns with genital ambiguity should have an adequate karyotype. Mixed gonadal dysgenesis is the second most common cause of genital ambiguity in the newborn. Because chromosome mosaicism is not unusual in intersex disorders, a thorough search for more than one cell line should be carried out. Buccal smears are not recommended because newborn infants with 46,XX karyotypes often have a low percentage of chromatin-positive cells until 2 weeks of life. Also, X chromatin bodies may be present in mosaics with Y chromosomal material. In intersex states there is often the need to clarify the origin of certain suspect sex chromosome fragments that are ambiguous with standard cytogenetics. DNA screening with a Y centromere probe may be helpful in such instances. High-resolution chromosome banding may be used to verify specific genetic syndromes such as Prader-Willi syndrome, where small deletions on the long arm of chromosome 15 have been identified in 50% of the cases.

Androgens

Androgen levels may be helpful to rule out maternal hyperandrogenism. Total testosterone, 17-hydroxyprogesterone, and dehydroepiandrosterone sulfate should be obtained from the mother in the delivery room. Defective androgen biosynthesis or lack of end organ sensitivity to androgen may lead to undermasculinization of male newborns (Figure 12-1). Usually these infants will have at least one palpable gonad on newborn physical examination. When the karyotype is 46,XY, basal levels of serum androstenediol, Δ^4-androstenedione, total testosterone, and dehydrotestosterone should be determined. If these levels are normal, repeated studies

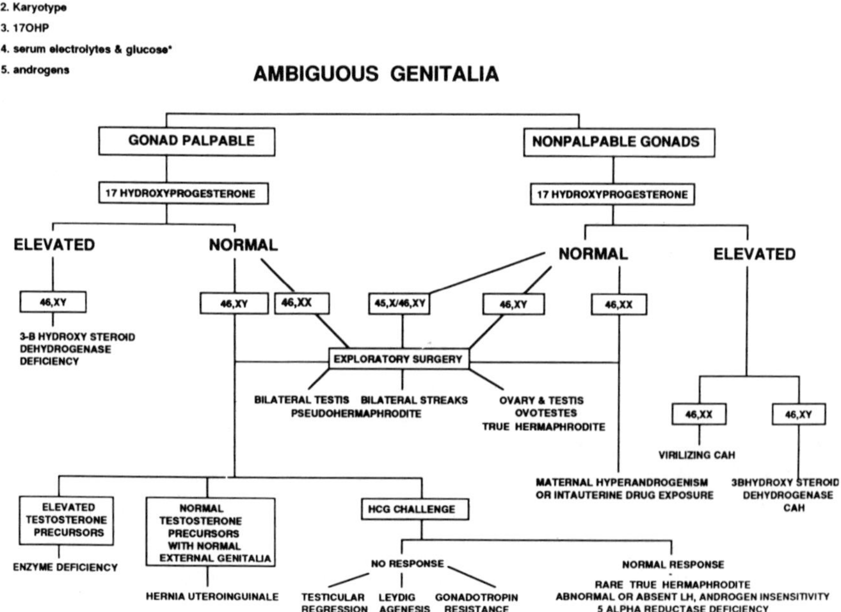

FIGURE 12-1. Flow chart for evaluating newborns with genital ambiguity. Sex assignment should not be given until all of the laboratory results are in and adequate consultation with specialists experienced in this area has been obtained. *If hypoglycemia is present the infant must be evaluated for congenital hypopituitarism.

after intramuscular human chorionic gonadotropin challenge may be helpful. It should be noted that these results are frequently equivocal in the peripartum period. Additionally, cross-reactivity of androgens in various assay systems may make such analysis impractical in the primary care setting. A capable reference laboratory must be identified. From a practical perspective, a phallus that appears reasonably adequate at birth may not be capable of responding to androgen at puberty. This fact must be considered when the gender assignment is made. For example, the 46,XY infant with genital ambiguity, a normal baseline androgen profile, and nonpalpable gonads can have incomplete testicular feminization, mixed gonadal dysgenesis, be a rare true hermaphrodite, or have 5-α-reductase deficiency. The sex of rearing should be female, however, because these individuals have no potential for reproductive function, female genital reconstruction is easier, and successful penile function cannot be guaranteed. Gonadectomy will be necessary to prevent potential virilization at puberty and the propensity toward gonadal malignancy.

Suggested Reading

Cassorla FG, Chrousos GP. Congenital adrenal hyperplasia. In: Becker KL, ed. Principles and practice of endocrinology and metabolism. Philadelphia: JB Lippincott, 1990:604–613.

Hung W. Micropenis, hypospadias, and cryptorchidism in infancy and childhood. In: Becker KL, ed. Principles and practice of endocrinology and metabolism. Philadelphia: JB Lippincott, 1990:760–766.

Jeffs RD, Gearhart JP. Reconstructive surgery of the male external genitalia. Semin Reprod Endocrinol 1987;5:315–326.

Mastroyannis C, Wallach EE. Male pseudohermaphroditism: inborn errors in testosterone biosynthesis. Semin Reprod Endocrinol 1987;5:261–276.

McDonough PG. Cytogenetics in reproductive endocrinology. In: Yen SCC, Jaffe RB, eds. Reproductive endocrinology, 3d ed. Philadelphia: WB Saunders, 1991: 462–479.

Oxford Monographs on Medical Genetics no. 27. Human malformations and related anomalies. Oxford: Oxford University Press, 1993.

Rhinedollar RH, Gray MR. The molecular basis of 21-hydroxylase deficiency. Semin Reprod Endocrinol 1991;9:34–45.

Rhinedollar RH, Tho SPT, McDonough PG. Abnormalities of sexual differentiation: evaluation and management. Clin Obstet Gynecol 1987;30:697–713.

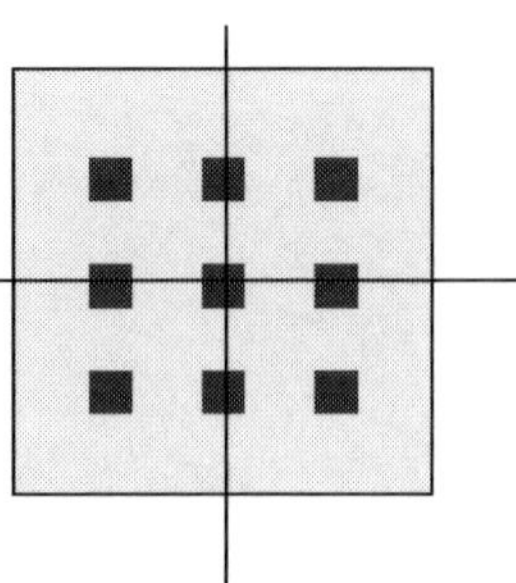

PART FOUR
Gynecology

13.
Vulvovaginitis

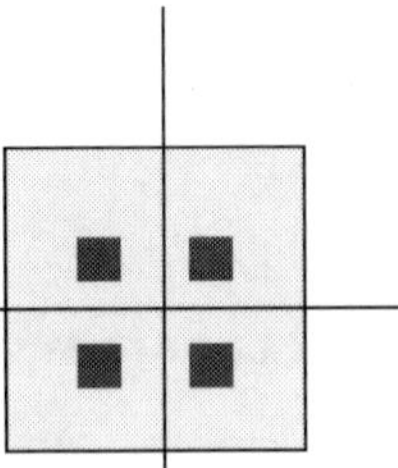

J. L. Thomason
P. J. Osypowski
J. A. James
N. J. Scaglione

Although not considered life threatening, vulvovaginitis is a serious problem often causing discomfort to women. Three infectious etiologies accounting for over 90% of vaginitides include bacterial vaginosis, vulvovaginal yeasts, and trichomoniasis. Office laboratory testing of vaginal secretions is the principle method of diagnosis for these conditions. This chapter discusses specimen collection and laboratory testing for women presenting with symptoms of vulvovaginitis.

Specimen Collection

Vaginal secretions should be obtained with a swab from the lateral vaginal walls, *not* the cul-de-sac or cervix. Specimens from women who have recently douched, used over the counter medications, or who have had recent intercourse are more difficult to evaluate. Douching causes dilutional effects, and recent intercourse elevates the vaginal pH.

Office Testing

Testing of vaginal secretions uses gross examination, pH measurement, testing for odor, and microscopic slide examination. Slide preparations of secretions mixed with physiologic saline and 10% KOH are prepared. An adequate saline slide preparation should have at least 15 vaginal squamous cells per low power field. KOH allows for identification of the amine odor associated with bacterial vaginosis and helps in the identification of yeast forms. Having pH paper with a range of 4.0–7.0 is additionally useful for the diagnosis of certain vaginitides.

Normal Laboratory Findings

Physiologic vaginal discharge usually appears flocculent rather than homogeneous and has no consistent odor associated with it. Women can misinterpret an excessive normal floccular discharge as the curdlike pattern of a yeast infection. The pH of normal vaginal secretions is ≤ 4.5. The vaginal squamous epithelial cells in normal women have few attached bacteria. The bacterial flora in normal women contains many lactobacillus morphotypes: long rods commonly referred to as Döederlein's bacilli.

Bacterial Vaginosis

Bacterial vaginosis is a polymicrobial disease with symptoms of copious, foul-smelling vaginal discharge. The predominating bacteria are obligate anaerobes (ie, *Bacteroides bivius, Bacteroides disiens, Mobiluncus* species, *Peptostreptococcus* species), microaerophilics (ie, *Mycoplasma hominis*), and facultative organisms (ie, *Gardnerella vaginalis*). Bacterial vaginosis has been associated with other infectious complications including salpingitis, dysfunctional uterine bleeding, chorioamnionitis, postpartum endometritis, preterm delivery, and postsurgical infections.

Office diagnosis of bacterial vaginosis can be made with the following findings:

1. Clue cells: vaginal epithelial cells so covered with attached bacteria that the borders of the cells are no longer clearly discernible
2. Fishlike odor on alkalinization of the secretions with KOH
3. Vaginal pH > 4.5
4. *Gardnerella* and anaerobic morphotypes exceeding lactobacilli morphotypes
5. Homogeneous vaginal discharge.

Strongest predictors of bacterial vaginosis are clue cells and odor.

Yeast Vulvovaginitis

Dense curdlike discharge, erythema, and pruritus occur in classic presentations of yeast vulvovaginitis, but many cases present with subtler findings. The best way to diagnose yeast infections is by wet mount analysis of vaginal secretions or vulvar specimens (skin scrapes). The saline suspension should be prepared and examined as previously described. In addition, a suspension of secretions in 10% KOH should be examined. This lyzes red cells, squamous cells, and leukocytes and leaves fungal elements intact. The finding of hyphal structures is pathognomonic for *Candida albicans*. The finding of only blastospores (buds) is less clear. Round to oval forms can be seen in the more rarely found *Candida glabrata*. The pH in patients with yeast infections is normal.

Trichomoniasis

Trichomonas vaginalis is an anaerobic, flagellated protozoan that causes sexually transmitted vulvovaginitis. The classically described green frothy foul-smelling discharge is found in < 5% of cases. Motile trichomonads can be easily visualized in saline wet mounts of vaginal secretions. In cases where the wet mount preparation is negative but trichomoniasis remains a possibility due to history or unexplained leukocytosis, a culture can be performed.

To culture for trichomonads, a swab containing vaginal secretions should be placed into modified Diamond's medium. This anaerobic liquid medium allows for growth of the protozoan when incubated at 35°C for 48–96 hours.

Atrophic Vulvovaginitis

For women lacking estrogen, vulvovaginal complaints may include thin watery discharge in addition to urinary problems and dyspareunia. Wet mount analysis of vaginal secretions shows increased parabasal cells, few if any lactobacilli, and a vaginal pH of 6.0–7.0. The other vaginitides should be ruled out.

Other Testing

Excessive amounts of leukocytes can be seen in a number of conditions including cervicitis, trichomoniasis, and erosive lichen planus. Bacterial vaginosis typically does not show excessive leukocytes.

Pap smear reports may include information regarding the presence of yeast and trichomonas. Yeast organisms are quite characteristic on the cytology smear. Trichomonads may sometimes be overcalled. Fragmented anucleate cells may sometimes be misinterpreted as the organism. The present Bethesda classification allows for notation on the cytology report that there is a shift in the bacterial flora (a paucity of lactobacillus morphotype). Cells with borders obscured by heavy coatings of bacteria can be readily identified. Although Pap smears can provide information regarding organisms associated with vulvovaginitis, it is not considered to be a diagnostic test to use when the patient presents with symptoms.

The clinical information obtained from vaginal cultures can be limited. In many cases the report returns with normal vaginal flora. Cultures from asymptomatic women will sometimes show yeast and gardnerella. It is better for the clinician to develop a more meticulous wet mount examination in the office. Rapid, in-office tests are currently being developed to supplement the health care professional who has limited microscopic examination experience.

Suggested Readings

Centers for Disease Control. 1989 Sexually transmitted diseases treatment guidelines. MMWR 1989;38(suppl 8):34–37.

Kaufman RH, Hammill HA. Vaginitis. Prim Care 1990;17:115–125.

Sobel JD. Vaginal infection in adult women. Med Clin North Am 1990;74:1573–1602.

Thomason JL, Gelbart SM. *Trichomonas vaginalis*. Obstet Gynecol 1989;74:536–541.

Thomason JL, Gelbart SM, Broekhuizen FF. Advances in the understanding of bacterial vaginosis. J Reprod Med 1989;34:581–587.

Thomason JL, Gelbart SM, Anderson RJ, Walt AK, Osypowski PJ, Broekhuizen FF. Statistical evaluation of diagnostic criteria for bacterial vaginosis. Am J Obstet Gynecol 1990;162:155–160.

14.
Upper Genital Tract Infection

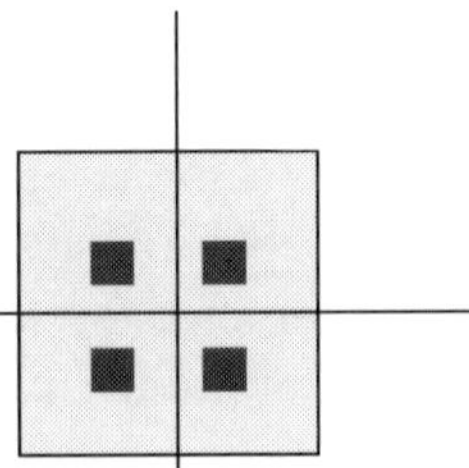

Susan Marie Mou

Upper genital tract infections may be caused by the ascent of microorganisms from the vagina and endocervix to the endometrium, fallopian tubes, ovaries, and adjacent structures, and, also, but less likely, by hematogenous or lymphatic spread, and rarely by direct injury to pelvic organs through surgery. The clinical laboratory evaluation of patients with upper genital infections is discussed in this chapter.

Blood Studies

A white cell count, differential, sedimentation rate, and C-reactive protein are usually ordered in patients presenting with symptoms of upper genital tract infection. However, these results can be variable and must be used carefully in conjunction with the patient's history, physical findings, and other laboratory and imaging studies. Significant elevation of these laboratory parameters may allow further testing to monitor treatment response, but as a rule, the patient's clinical response is key to evaluation of disease resolution.

Blood cultures are rarely positive, but may be considered in some patients with fevers ≥ 38.5°C, where the return of positive cultures will be higher. Blood culture yield is higher in septic abortions than in other pelvic infections (1). Pregnancy testing is important to rule out ectopic pregnancy. Salpingitis and ectopic pregnancy may coexist (2). Serologic testing has a limited role in the laboratory evaluation of upper genital tract infections. Serum chlamydial IgG and IgM titers may rise fourfold in females with an acute infection due to *Chlamydia* organisms, but cervical screening for chlamydia is more quickly available for diagnosis. Serologic studies are hampered by the need for serial testing (delayed results) and by the high background positivity in the sexually active population.

Gram Stain

The presence of gram-negative intracellular diplococci on Gram stain of cervical secretions is helpful only for positive slides and predicts *Neisseria gonorrhoeae* infection in only 60% of women, as compared to 95% of men (3). Gram-negative diplococci representing other types of *Neisseria* organisms can lead to false positive results. Culturing or DNA probes are more helpful in the diagnosis. A Gram stain of endocervical discharge showing > 5–10 leukocytes per oil immersion field is thought by some to be suspicious for chlamydia infection (4). This may not be reliable in pregnancy. If a clostridial infection is suspected in an upper genital tract infection, the Gram stain may be helpful in identification of large gram-positive bacilli.

Organism Identification

Traditional culture isolation and identification have been augmented or replaced by numerous rapid and sensitive techniques using immunoassays and DNA probes. Specimens used in the evaluation of upper genital tract infections may be obtained from the cervix, peritoneal fluid (culdocentesis or laparoscopy), abscess fluid or tissue, and endometrial aspirates.

Cervical evaluation has traditionally been performed for patients with upper genital tract infections. Correlation does not always exist between cervical organisms and those obtained by laparoscopy. Laboratory studies of the cervix primarily focus on identification of *N gonorrhoeae* and *Chlamydia trachomatis*. *N gonorrhoeae* may be diagnosed by a culture or DNA probe specimen of the endocervix. *C trachomatis* may be identified by different methods, including DNA probe, culture, enzyme immunoassay, and fluorescent antibody.

In patients undergoing laparoscopy, cultures should be obtained from the fallopian tubes for anaerobic bacteria, facultative bacteria, *N gonorrhoeae*, and *C trachomatis*. The cul-de-sac fluid can be cultured for anaerobic and facultative bacteria and *N gonorrhoeae*. Because chlamydia is an obligate, intracellular organism cul-de-sac fluid is not optimal for culture. Rapid tests for *C trachomatis* may be falsely positive due to anaerobic bacteria and enteric bacteria, so should not be used on peritoneal fluid.

Fimbrial biopsy for pathologic and microbiologic evaluation is advocated by some (2,5) and does not appear to increase adhesive disease postoperatively. If an abscess is present, the abscess wall obtained at surgery is the best site for culture.

Culdocentesis may allow the clinician to obtain purulent material from an abscess or the peritoneal cavity from which cultures and Gram stain can be performed. Obtaining clear fluid may help to rule out pelvic inflammatory disease. The culdocentesis results are limited by vaginal contamination (6). In postoperative patients a less optimal culture site is the vaginal cuff; this can only give information on what vaginal flora are present. Only aerobic cultures should be obtained from vaginal cuff material.

Endometrial Biopsy

An endometrial biopsy or aspirate can be obtained and cultured for *N gonorrhoeae, C trachomatis,* and anaerobic and facultative bacteria. Correlation with laparoscopy is high, with an 84% positive predictive value in the diagnosis of pelvic inflammatory disease confirmed by laparoscopy as shown by Paavonen and colleagues (7). Histologic specimens from endometrial biopsies showing five or more neutrophils per 400× field in endometrial surface epithelium and one or more plasma cells per 120× field in the endometrial stroma have been shown to be 92% sensitive and 87% specific as compared to laparoscopically confirmed acute salpingitis (8).

Laboratory Screening to Prevent Infections

Patients undergoing abortion-related procedures should be screened for chlamydia and gonorrhea, preferably before the procedure. Full treatment doses of tetracycline or doxycycline need to be given to chlamydia-positive women. Women with *C trachomatis* cervical infection at the time of abortion are at increased risk for postabortal endometritis or salpingitis or both. Approximately 23% to 38% of women with *C trachomatis* cervicitis versus 2% to 10% of those negative for *C trachomatis* develop postpartum pelvic infection (9). Bacterial vaginosis has also been implicated as a marker for increased postabortal infections (10).

References

1. Rotheram EB, Schick SF. Nonclostridial anaerobic bacteria in septic abortion. Am J Med 1969;46:80.
2. Sellors J, Mahony J, Goldsmith C, et al. The accuracy of clinical findings and

laparoscopy for pelvic inflammatory disease. Am J Obstet Gynecol 1991; 164:113–120.

3. Sweet R, Gibbs R. Infectious diseases of the female genital tract. Baltimore: Williams & Wilkins, 1985:2.

4. Brunham RC, Paavonen J, Stevens CE, et al. Mucopurulent cervicitis: the ignored counterpart in women of urethritis in men. N Engl J Med 1984; 311:1–7.

5. Soper D. Diagnosis and laparoscopic grading of acute salpingitis. Am J Obstet Gynecol 1991;164:1370–1376.

6. Sweet RL, Draper DL, Schachter J, et al. Microbiology and pathogenesis of acute salpingitis as determined by laparoscopy: What's the appropriate site to sample? Am J Obstet Gynecol 1980;138:985–989.

7. Paavonen J, Aine R, Teisala K, et al. Comparison of endometrial biopsy and peritoneal fluid cytologic testing with laparoscopy in the diagnosis of acute pelvic inflammatory disease. Am J Obstet Gynecol 1985;151:645–650.

8. Kiviat NB, Wolner-Hanssen P, Eschenbach DA, et al. Endometrial histopathology in patients with culture-proved upper genital tract infection and laparoscopically diagnosed acute salpingitis. Am J Surg Pathol 1990;14:167–175.

9. McGregor JA. Chlamydial infection in women. Obstet Gynecol Clin North Am 1989;16:565–592.

10. Larson PG, Krohn MA, Klebanoff SJ, et al. Incidence of pelvic inflammatory disease after first-trimester legal abortion in women with bacterial vaginosis after treatment with metronidazole: a double-blind, randomized study. Am J Obstet Gynecol 1992;166:100–103.

15.
Sexual Assault

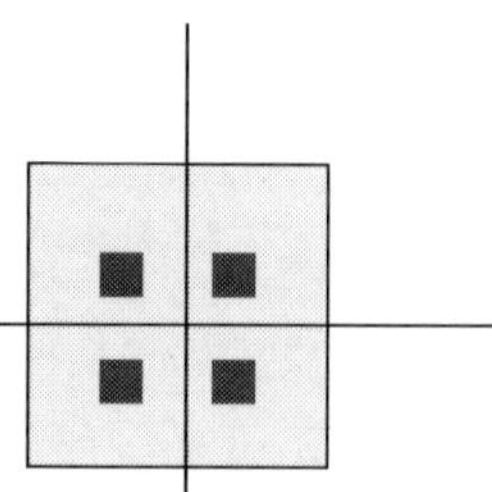

Bonnie Dattel

It is estimated that only 10% to 33% of all sexual assault cases are reported; however, over 81,000 cases per year are treated by medical personnel (1). Proper medical treatment in sexual assault cases requires attention to trauma, infectious disease complications, forensic evidence, and the emotional needs of the victim. This chapter focuses on the clinical laboratory's role in the evaluation of sexual assault.

Forensic Evidence

The collection of forensic evidence in instances of sexual assault is of utmost importance to the successful prosecution of these cases. Careful attention to the details involved in the collection of materials for forensic evaluation as well as their proper handling are mandatory. Evidence collection falls into two categories. One involves the collection of "trace" evidence (ie., hairs, blood traces, debris, etc), and the second involves evaluation for the presence of seminal fluid from sites of assault. Forensic tests are listed in Table 15-1, and a more specific guide to specimen collection is found in Table 15-2.

Pubic and head hair is transferred between persons after close contact. Clothing, pubic hair combings, and other hairs noted on the body of the victim are submitted for analysis. Examination of hairs includes evaluation of their length, relative diameter, color, and degree of curl or curve (2). Questioned hairs are mounted for microscopic comparison and undergo polymerase chain reaction (PCR) typing of the hair root (3). In general,

TABLE 15-1. Evaluation in sexual assault

Forensic Evidence	*Other*
Trace Evidence	Toxicology
Outerwear	Pregnancy testing
Underwear	Initial and 2 wk
Head hair combings (victim)	Blood typing (victim)
Pubic hair combings (victim)	Can be done at follow-up
Wood's lamp fluorescence	Saliva (victim)
	Hair samples with follicles (victim)
Antigen	
P-30	
Enzymes	
Acid Phosphatase	
Peptidase A	
PGM-I	
Semen	
Microscopic slide for motility	
(normal saline)	
DNA fingerprinting	
PCR/DNA fingerprinting	

results from hair analyses have reported a low incidence of significant pubic hair transfers from suspect to victim. Significant head hair transfers can occur on outerwear.

Additional trace evidence that can be obtained from clothing includes grasses, other plant matter, dirt, sand, and fibers from vehicles or carpet materials. Sealed evidence containers of porous material help to prevent bacterial or fungal overgrowth.

Although rape law does not require that emission has occurred, the recognition of semen in collected samples for criminal evidence is clearly important. Samples from reported areas of assault are taken with sterile cotton-tipped swabs, gently rolled in normal saline on a slide, and coverslipped. Microscopic evaluation is performed for sperm identification and evidence of sperm motility. Additional air-dried slides are also prepared for later analysis of seminal enzymes. Acid phosphatase can be eluted either directly from biologic site specimens or seminal stains from clothing (4). Additional tests that can be performed on seminal fluid include ABO and

TABLE 15-2. Guide to specimen collection in sexual assault cases

Clinical Specimens for Hospital or Reference Laboratory	Evidence Collection	Evidence for Crime Laboratory
		All swabs and slides must be thoroughly air dried before packaging. Code corresponding swabs and slides, eg, oral swab #1, oral slide #1.
	Note condition of clothing on arrival. Collect outer and underclothing worn during or immediately after assault. Collect fingernail scrapings if indicated.	Clothing (in separate paper bags) Foreign materials on clothing Fingernail scrapings
	Conduct general physical exam. Scan entire body with Wood's lamp. Collect dried and moist secretions and foreign materials from body including head, hair, and scalp. Document findings.	Dried secretions Foreign materials
Base line GC culture from oropharynx. Take other STD cultures as indicated	Examine oral cavity for injury. Document findings if indicated by history. Swab area around mouth. Collect 2 oral swabs up to 6 hs postassault and prepare 2 dry mount slides. Take specimen for GC culture.	Dried secretions 2 swabs from oral cavity 2 dry mount slides 1 swab from area around mouth
	Examine external genitalia for injury. Scan with Wood's lamp. Collect dried and moist secretions and foreign materials. Document findings. Cut matted pubic	Dried secretions Foreign materials Matted pubic hair cuttings Pubic hair combings Comb

TABLE 15-2, continued

Clinical Specimens for Hospital or Reference Laboratory	*Evidence Collection*	*Evidence for Crime Laboratory*
	hair. Comb pubic hair to collect foreign materials.	
Base line GC culture from endocervix. Take other STD cultures as indicated	Examine vagina and cervix for injury and foreign materials. Collect 3 swabs from vaginal pool. Prepare 1 wet mount slide and 2 dry mount slides. Examine wet mount for sperm. Document findings. Collect cervical swabs only if assault occurred more than 24 hs prior to exam and no possibility exists of contaminating specimen from previous coitus. Take specimen for GC culture.	Foreign materials 3 vaginal swabs 1 wet mount slide 2 dry mount slides Aspirate/washings for sperm optional
Base line GC culture from rectum. Take other STD cultures as indicated	Examine buttocks, perianal skin, and anal folds for injury. Collect dried and moist secretions and foreign materials. Document findings if indicated by history and/or findings: collect 2 rectal swabs and prepare 2 dry mount slides. Take specimen for GC culture. Conduct an anoscopic or proctoscopic exam if rectal injury is suspected.	Dried secretions Foreign materials 2 rectal swabs 2 dry mount slides
Syphilis and pregnancy base line	Clinical tests. Pregnancy test—blood (red top tube) or urine. Syphilis serology (red top tube).	

TABLE 15-2, continued

Clinical Specimens for Hospital or Reference Laboratory	Evidence Collection	Evidence for Crime Laboratory
	Other evidence collected at discretion of physician and law enforcement officer. Patient has the right to refuse these tests. Blood alcohol/toxicology (grey top tube). Urine toxicology screen (urine specimen).	Alcohol/tox samples
	Reference samples can be collected at time of exam or at later date according to local crime laboratory procedures. Blood typing (yellow top tube). Saliva specimen. 15–20 head hairs. 15–20 pubic hairs.	Reference samples
Clinical specimens to hospital or reference laboratory		Evidence to law enforcement officer for crime laboratory

Adapted from state of California Medical Protocol

ABH grouping, HLA typing, secretor status, P-30 antigen, phosphoglucomutase, and peptidase A (5,6; see also Part 7).

Other laboratory analyses in the evaluation of sexual assault include pregnancy testing at initial and follow-up examinations and toxicology screening (urine and blood) in cases where the victim states that unknown substances were part of the assault.

Perhaps the newest and most exciting technique in criminal investigations is assailant identification from semen by DNA fingerprinting techniques (7). Coupled with PCR, DNA techniques can allow assistant identification from extremely small amounts of material, such as a few spermatozoa.

In regard to collection of specimens for semen analysis the following points are emphasized:

1. The yield from oropharyngeal samples is markedly reduced after 6 hours (6).
2. Caution must be exercised if specimens are obtained from the endocervical canal due to the long period of time from which spermatozoa can be identified from this site (up to 17 days, nonmotile).
3. Although most centers use an arbitrary time frame of 72 hours for collection of forensic evidence, semen may be retrieved from the vagina as long as 7 days after the assault.
4. In general, for vagina specimens a range of 30 minutes to 3 hours has been accepted as the period during which motile sperm are most likely to be recovered.
5. Rectal specimens are best collected through an anoscope to avoid contamination from vaginal "run down."
6. A Wood's lamp may be of help in identifying seminal fluid "fluorescence."

Assessment for Sexually Transmitted Disease

Microbiologic specimens evaluated in cases of sexual assault are listed in Table 15-3. Cultures for *Neisseria gonorrhoeae* should be taken from all sites involved in the assault (ie, pharyngeal, cervical, rectal) and plated on Thayer-Martin media for isolation. Cultures for *Chlamydia trachomatis* at the time of initial evaluation are controversial because if *C trachomatis* is identified within several hours of the assault, it most likely was a preexisting condition due to the longer incubation required for this obligate intracellular organism (8). Acceptable methods for identification of *C trachomatis* include direct staining with fluorescein-labeled monoclonal antibody and culture by microtiter plate method or cyclohexamide-treated McCoy cells in monolayers (9).

Cultures for other sexually transmitted diseases (STDs), such as viral infections, are generally unwarranted at the time of initial evaluation. Culture with Feinberg-Whittington media for both *Candida* and *Trichomonas* organisms are acceptable; however, the microscopic evaluation of discharge (saline and KOH preparations) from the vagina or urethra is as sensitive as culture technique for the identification of these organisms and much more cost effective.

Cultures and microscopic evaluation of vaginal discharge should be repeated within 2 weeks after the initial evaluation, as well. This follow-up examination will allow the documentation of the acquisition of STDs as well

TABLE 15-3. Microbiologic specimens in cases of sexual assault

Cultures

Thayer-Martin Media	*N gonorrhoeae*	Initial and follow-up
Cyclohexamide treated	*C trachomatis*	Only if clinically
McCoy cells		suspect
Feinberg-Whittington	Candida, trichomonas	

Wet Mount

Normal saline	BV (Bacterial vaginosis),	Initial and 2-wk
10% KOH	trichomonas	follow-up
	Candida	

Colposcopy/Cytology

	HPV Human papilloma virus	Initial and 8-wk
	HSV Herpes Simplex virus	follow-up

Serologies

VDRL or MHA-TP	Syphilis	Paired initial and
Hepatitis B		6–8-wk follow-up
HIV		
IgG, IgM	Chlamydia	

as their treatment. Data suggest that it is the follow-up examination that is most important in documentation of disease acquisition from assault (10).

Certain STDs are not easily identified by culture, but rather require serologic evaluation to confirm their acquisition. The serologic evaluation must be done in two phases. First, a serum sample obtained at the time of initial intake should be obtained for syphilis (VDRL or microhemagglutination-*Treponema pallidum* [MHA-TP]), human immunodeficiency virus (HIV) antibody and hepatitis B serology. This initial serum sample must be paired with a second sample obtained at least 8 weeks later to differentiate infection that was preexisting from that which is newly acquired.

Acquisition of HIV infection from sexual assault is of primary concern for many survivors, and for some (up to 20%) it is their sole reason for coming forward for medical evaluation (11). There is little data to suggest that sexual assault is a high risk even for HIV seroconversion (12). Anecdotal reports exist documenting that sexual assault was the only mode of infection for certain individuals (13). The issue of HIV infection must be approached with great sensitivity and should include patient education and individual risk assessment at the time of initial consent for antibody testing. The risk of false positives is low, particularly when the standard enzyme-linked immunosorbent assay is coupled with Western blot analysis (14).

Hepatitis B, herpes simplex virus (HSV), and human papillomavirus (HPV) are potential viral infections that could occur following sexual assault; however, few data exist regarding the incidence in survivors. Colposcopy and cytology may be helpful in the evaluation of HSV and HPV.

References

1. Glaser JB, Hammerschlag MR, McCormack WM. Epidemiology of sexually transmitted diseases in rape victims. Rev Infect Dis 1989;2:246–254.
2. Mann M-J. Hair transfers in sexual assault: a six year case study. J Forens Sci 1990;35:951–955.
3. Scochetman G, Ou C-Y, Jones WK. Polymerase chain reaction. J Infect Dis 1988;158:1154–1157.
4. Kind SS. The acid phosphatase test. In: Curry AS, ed. Methods of forensic science, vol III. London: Interscience, 1965:267–288.
5. Sensabaugh GF. Isolation and characterization of a semen-specific protein from human seminal plasma: a potential new marker for semen identification. J Forens Sci 1978;23:106–115.
6. Baechtel FS. In: Saferstein R, ed. Forensic science handbook, vol II. Englewood Cliffs: Prentice-Hall, 1988: 348–382.
7. Honma M, Yoshiu T, Ishiyama I, et al. Individual identification from semen by the deoxyribonucleic acid (DNA) fingerprint technique. J F S C A 1989;34:222–227.
8. Schachter J, Dattel BJ. Sexually transmitted diseases in victims of sexual assault. New Engl J Med 1987;316:1023–1024.
9. Ripka KT, Marder P. A cultivation of *Chlamydia trachomatis* in cyclohexamide-treated McCoy cells. J Clin Microbiol 1977;6:3288.
10. Jenny CJ, Hooton TM, Bowers A, et al. Sexually transmitted disease in victims of rape. N Engl J Med 1990;322:713–716.
11. Estsreich S, Forster GE, Robinson A. Sexually transmitted diseases in rape victims. Genitourin Med 1990;66:433–438.
12. DiGiovanni C, Berlin F, Casterella P, et al. Prevalence of HIV antibody among a group of paraphilic sex offenders. J Acquire Immune Defic Syndr 1991; 4:633–637.
13. Murphy S, Kitchen V, Harris JRW, et al. Rape and subsequent seroconversion to HIV. Br Med J 1989;2299:718.
14. Schwartz JS, Dans PE, Kinosian BP. Human immunodeficiency virus test evaluation, performance and uses—proposals to make good tests better. JAMA 1988;259:2574–2579.

16.
Urine Evaluation

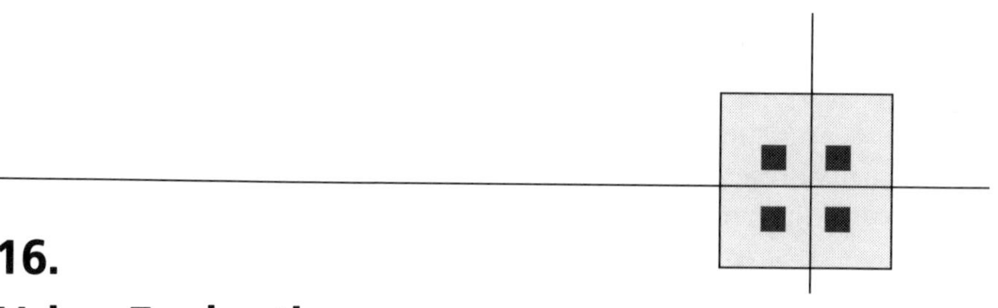

Nicolette Horbach

This chapter discusses the clinical laboratory evaluation of urinary tract infections (UTIs) and routine urinalysis. Additional information regarding UTIs in pregnancy can be found in Chapter 5.

Acute Urinary Tract Infections

Approximately 25% of women experience an acute UTI each year, resulting in millions of office visits to primary care physicians. Women are particularly susceptible to cystitis because of their anatomically short urethra and the extensive colonization of the vaginal introitus with uropathogens from the rectal reservoir. Diaphragm users are prone to infections, which may be partially due to obstruction of the urethra or urethral trauma caused by the diaphragm. Recent evidence also implicates vaginal spermicides in the pathogenesis of coitally related UTIs due to changes in the vaginal pH and normal bacterial flora. The primary pathogen in community-acquired infections is *Escherichia coli* (80%) although recent reports have indicated that 10% to 20% of acute infections in young women are due to *Staphylococcus saprophyticus*. Other pathogens include *Klebsiella* species, *Proteus* species, *Enterobacter* species, *Pseudomonas aeruginosa*, and *Streptococcus fecalis*.

In patients with an initial UTI, a presumptive diagnosis may be made in a symptomatic patient if the microscopic urinalysis of a clean catch midstream urine specimen reveals bacteria and white blood cells or a positive leukocyte and nitrite test is obtained on dipstick evaluation.

Empiric treatment may be started in this circumstance without a urine culture. Culture and sensitivities should be performed if the patient has a history of a recent UTI, symptoms of a UTI for more than 5 days, persistent symptoms while taking antibiotics, recent urinary tract instrumentation or surgery, or diabetes. Assistance in obtaining a clean catch can be provided to obese patients by asking the patient to void while on an examination room table with stirrups. A catheterized urine specimen should be obtained when midstream clean catch specimens yield repetitively contaminated samples.

Laboratory diagnosis of UTIs uses microscopic evaluations of unspun urine and sediment following centrifugation, dipstick evaluation of nitrite and leukocyte esterase, and culture methods.

The microscopic evaluation of an unspun urine specimen should reveal one or more bacteria per high power field if there are $> 10^4$ colony-forming units (cfu) of bacteria per mL of urine. Pyuria is defined as > 10 leukocytes/per mL in unspun urine and should be present in nearly all women with acute UTIs. Pyuria can also be found in women with a negative urine culture due to chlamydial urethritis. Microscopic hematuria is seen in approximately 50% of women with acute cystitis and is rarely found in other conditions associated with noninfectious dysuria.

An alternative to urine microscopy is the urine dipstick test for leukocyte esterase and nitrites. The urinary nitrite test detects the conversion of urinary nitrate to nitrite by bacteria within the bladder. The esterase test is a colorometric evaluation that detects the presence of esterase within leukocytes in the urine. To optimize the accuracy of these tests, they should be performed on a concentrated first morning void. False negative results may be obtained if the specimen is collected at other times, in patients with infections due to enterococci because they do not convert nitrate to nitrite, and in the presence of urinary dyes such as phenazopyridine (Pyridium®) or bilirubin.

Urinary cultures have long been the primary tool used to diagnose acute UTIs. The traditional approach of defining a positive culture as more than 10^5 cfu mL urine has been questioned by several authors. Twenty to 24% of women with symptomatic infections will have $< 10^5$ cfu/mL urine. Important work by Stamm suggests that for symptomatic women, a bacterial count of 10^2 cfu/mL on urine culture should be sufficient to establish the diagnosis of an acute UTI, and treatment should be initiated.

Numerous antibiotic regimens have been advocated for the treatment of bacteriuria, and there has been significant debate regarding the optimal duration of therapy for the patient with an uncomplicated infection. Currently a significant body of literature exists supporting the use of single-dose antibiotic therapy in select women. This is nearly as effective in treating acute infections and preventing recurrent infections as the older 7-day courses of treatment while producing fewer side effects. Single-dose therapy is contraindicated in women with symptoms for more than 5 days, pregnancy, immunosuppression, renal tract anomalies, and indwelling catheters. Because symptoms of a UTI may persist for more than 24 hours, many clinicians use abbreviated 3- to 5-day treatments. The patient is asked to return to the laboratory in 7–10 days for follow-up urine cultures. Routine posttherapy test of cure cultures have also been debated. They may be helpful in distinguishing persistent infections and reinfection with new organisms in women with persistent or frequently recurring symptoms.

Routine Urinalysis

The components of urinalysis and the clinical correlates are listed in Table 16-1. Urinalysis evaluates macroscopic features (color, odor, etc), microscopic features (bacteria, white blood cells, casts, etc), and chemical analyses (dipstick). Screening urinalysis has the potential of detecting UTIs, neoplasms, renal disease, and diabetes in the asymptomatic patient although these tests are rarely positive. Use of dipstick analysis without the laboratory microscopic examination may offer a less expensive alternative for those who perform urinalysis screening examinations. Patients with a positive urine dipstick analysis should have confirmation of the abnormality by urine microscopy.

The finding of glucosuria should lead to evaluation of renal function if serum glucose levels are normal. Excessive urinary protein is indicative of UTI or renal dysfunction, but the clinician should be aware of the false positive results with dipstick analysis. Cystitis and contamination secondary to menses should initially be considered for women with evidence of hematuria. Cytologic examination may be a helpful adjunct in the evaluation of asymptomatic microhematuria in women. Voided sampling for urinary cytology will be more accurate if obtained after exercise or agitation of the bladder during a pelvic examination. Persistent microscopic hematuria requires a more thorough evaluation of the urinary tract. Bacteriuria may be asymptomatic, particularly in the elderly in whom bacteriuria is more prevalent than in younger women.

TABLE 16-1. Urinalysis—clinical correlates

Urinalysis (Dipstick Evaluation)	Clinical Correlates for Ob/Gyn
Urine pH (normal 4.5–8.0)	Alkaline urine suggests infection with urea-splitting organisms (ie, *Proteus mirabilis*)
Urine protein (dipstick is negative when level is < 100 mg/L	Proteinuria may be transient in some disorders or suggest the presence of a UTI
	Monitored in pregnancy to diagnose Preeclampsia
Urine glucose	Present with diabetes and altered renal threshold
Hemoglobin	May be of benefit in assessing for renal stones in the absence of bacteriuria
Nitrite test	Most of the common urinary pathogens reduce nitrates to nitrites; enterococcus is an exception
Leukocyte esterase	Released by polymorphonuclear cells in urine, helps to identify pyuria but affected by vaginal discharge
Ketones	May be helpful in evaluation of hyperemesis gravidarum; positive in diabetic ketoacidosis

Urinalysis (Microscopic Evaluation)	Clinical Correlates for Ob/Gyn
Cells	
Erythrocytes Leukocytes Bacteria Renal and transitional cells Squamous cells	Microscopic examination primarily helps in the evaluation of UTIs, urinary incontinence assessment of renal stone in patients with flank and lower abdominal pain. Patients with microscopic hematuria and a negative urine culture and sensitivity should be referred for urologic work-up (80% of patients will have an identifiable abnormality)
	Numerous squamous cells indicate vaginal contamination
Casts, Crystals	

Suggested Reading

Baldassarre JS, Kaye D. Special problems of urinary tract infection in the elderly. Med Clin North Am 1991;75:375–390.

Bard RH. The significance of asymptomatic microhematuria in women and its economic implications. Arch Intern Med 1988;148:2629–2632.

Bolann BJ, Sandberg S, Digranes A. Implications of probability analysis for interpreting results of leukocyte esterase and nitrite test strips. Clin Chem 1989; 35:1663–1668.

Bump RC. Urinary tract infection in women. Current role of single-dose therapy. J Reprod Med 1990;35:785–791.

Carel RS, Silverberg DS, Kaminsky R, et al. Routine urinalysis (dipstick) findings in mass screening of healthy adults. Clin Chem 1987;33:2106–2108.

Kiel DP, Moskowitz MA. The urinalysis: a critical appraisal. Med Clin North Am 1987;71:607–624.

Powers RD. New directions in the diagnosis and therapy of urinary tract infections. Am J Obstet Gynecol 1991;164:1387–1389.

Ronald AR, Conway B, Zhanel GG. The value of single-dose therapy to diagnose the site of urinary infection. Chemotherapy 1990;36(suppl 1):2–9.

Stamm WE, Counts GW, Running KR, et al. Diagnosis of coliform infection in acutely dysuric women. N Eng J Med 1982;307:463–482.

Thomas S, Bhatia NN. New approaches in the treatment of urinary tract infections. Obstet Gynecol Clin North Am 1989;16:897–909.

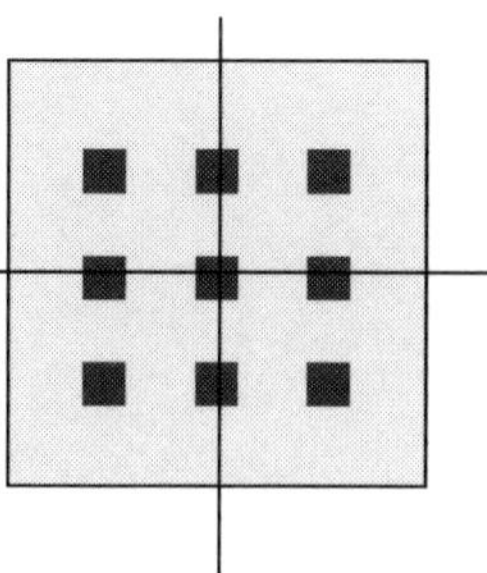

PART FIVE

Endocrinology and Infertility

17.
Hormone Analysis

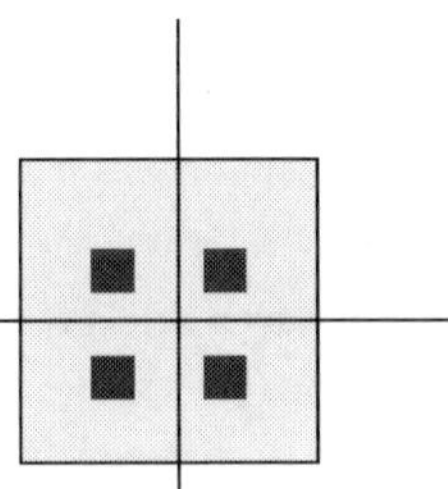

Kathy A. Trumbull
James A. Simon

The earliest method of measuring hormones was the bioassay, an indirect test that dealt with observing the effect of a biologic sample, which presumably contained a hormone, on a target organ. An early classic example of a bioassay is the ovarian change seen in rats or rabbits in response to human chorionic gonadotropin (hCG) in a pregnant woman's urine. Over the past 30 years, hormonal assay methods have changed significantly.

The two principle impediments to hormonal measurement have been the need for assays with sensitivities sufficient enough to measure hormones at the low concentrations at which they are normally circulating and assays with specificities such that reliable levels can be obtained in the presence of a wide variety of substances. We can now measure the concentrations of hormones in biologic samples directly with much greater sensitivity and precision. With the advent of the radioimmunoassay in 1960 came the ability to measure hormones present in biologic fluids in very small quantities, even below the nanogram (10^{-9}) and picogram range (10^{-12}). Precision has been aided by use of monoclonal antibodies.

Bioassay

Measurement of hormonal activity was less refined in the older in vivo bioassay methods where organ weight and histologic changes were the end points. An example of a newer in vitro bioassay is one where the measurement of testosterone production by dispersed rat Leydig cells is used to assess luteinizing hormone (LH) and hCG. This test is more sensitive but cannot distinguish between LH and the hCG because they both function through a common receptor. In most current clinical situations, in vivo and in vitro bioassays are rarely used. The bioassay has some role in the development of newer assays, but generally suffers in regard to specificity, sensitivity, precision, and cost.

Chemical Assays

The chemical methods of measuring hormones are based on reactions of steroids with specific compounds (evaluated by colorimetry or fluorometry) or separation methods such as chromatography. Like the bioassay, the use of chemical assays is limited, having been replaced by immunoassay techniques.

Most chemical assays involve urine as the specimen, which is usually available in large amounts and contains large amounts of the hormone or its metabolites. Many of these assays will not work with blood, or results are much less reliable because of the small amounts of hormone present. The assays require a considerable amount of processing and are time consuming.

Immunoassays

All types of immunoassays are based on the use of antibodies against the hormone. These antibodies are raised in various animals, such as mice or rabbits, against human hormones. When immunoassays were first developed, polyclonal antibodies were used. These antibodies often lacked specificity as evidenced by the significant cross-reactivity between hormonal substances (ie, LH and hCG). Specificity improved with the use of monoclonal antibodies and other modifications of the immunoassays.

Immunoassays can be divided into nonlabeled or labeled types. Nonlabeled assays include precipitin reactions, agglutination methods, and nephelometric (light scattering) analyses. Labeled assays use radioisotopes, enzymes, or luminescent compounds (fluorescent or chemiluminescent).

Immunoassays can either be competitive or noncompetitive. Competitive assays follow the law of mass action, with competition for sites by labeled and unlabeled substance. An example of the noncompetitive assay is the immunoradiometric assay. This type of assay requires two antibodies, both against the hormone, but at different sites. One antibody is attached to a solid phase, usually bound covalently. The other antibody is the labeled antibody. The hormone is caught between the antibodies, to form a "sandwich." Figures 17-1, 17-2, and 17-3 demonstrate schematically three different immunoassay methodologies.

Practical Points

Assays are inherently less accurate at the high or low ends of the scale. To quantify large amounts of the hormone present in a sample, dilutions must be made, which can be slightly inaccurate. The slight inaccuracy is then multiplied by virtue of the necessary calculations to arrive at the final value for the sample. On the low end of the assay, a relatively larger range of label represents a given quantity of unknown, thereby making it more difficult to interpret (Figure 17-4).

A standard is a known preparation. The standard hormone must be immunochemically identical to the unknown hormone being evaluated.

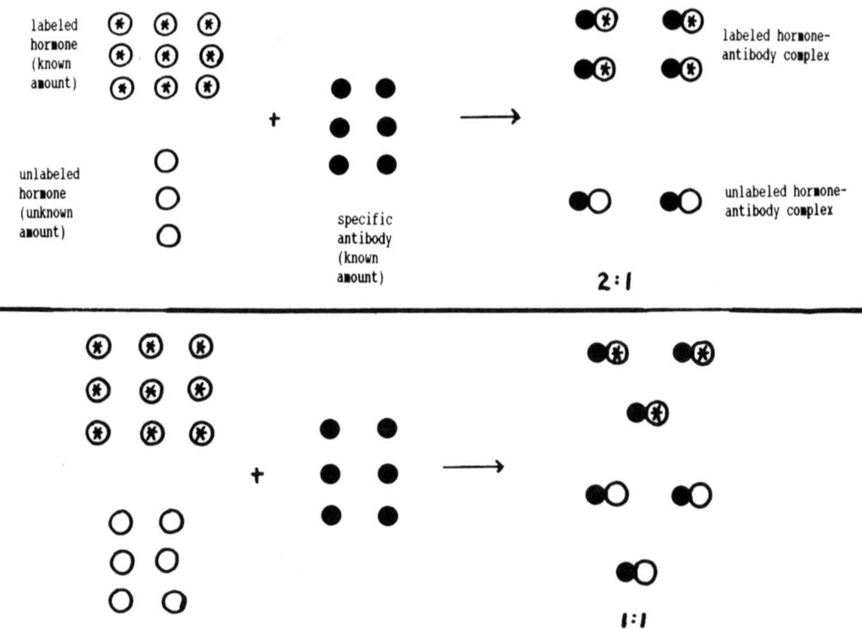

FIGURE 17-1. Competitive inhibition. As more unlabeled, unknown hormone is added to the reaction, the ratio of labeled hormone-antibody complex to unlabeled hormone-antibody complex decreases. The amount of labeled hormone bound to the antibodies will reflect the concentration of unlabeled hormone.

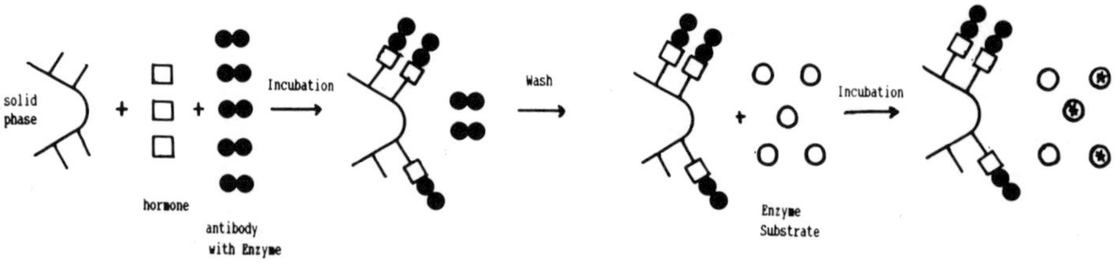

FIGURE 17-2. Enzyme immunoassay. After the hormone-antibody-enzyme complex is formed, the final step of incubation with enzyme substrate produces an "activated" substrate whose concentration will reflect the amount of hormone present.

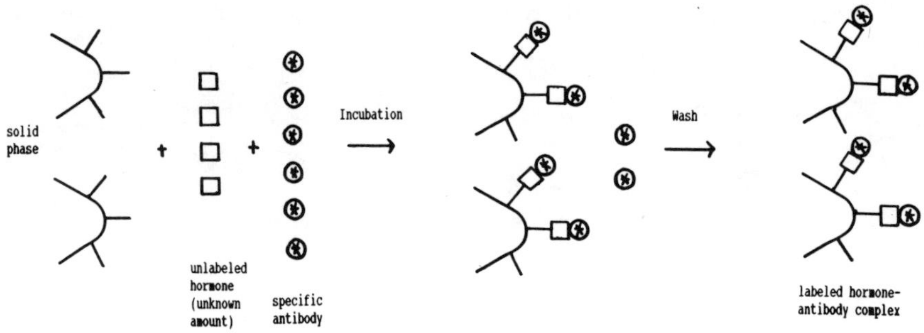

FIGURE 17-3. Immunoradiometric "sandwich" assay. The solid phase antibody attaches to the hormone at its specific site, thereby attaching the hormone to the solid phase. All hormone in the sample is attached to the solid phase. The second antibody binds to the hormone at its specific site, different from the first, so that a hormone "sandwich" is created between the two antibodies. After washing out excess antibody the label is quantified.

Steroids are available as pure chemical preparations, but peptide hormones are not. To be able to compare results between different laboratories, internationally accepted reference preparations have been developed. For some hormones such as prolactin, LH, follicle-stimulating hormone, and hCG, more than one international reference preparation is available. Thus, the interpretation of the results of an assay depends on which reference preparations are used in that specific laboratory. Physicians should know what reference preparations are in use at the laboratory of their choice.

It is customary to calculate the 95% confidence limits for the establish-

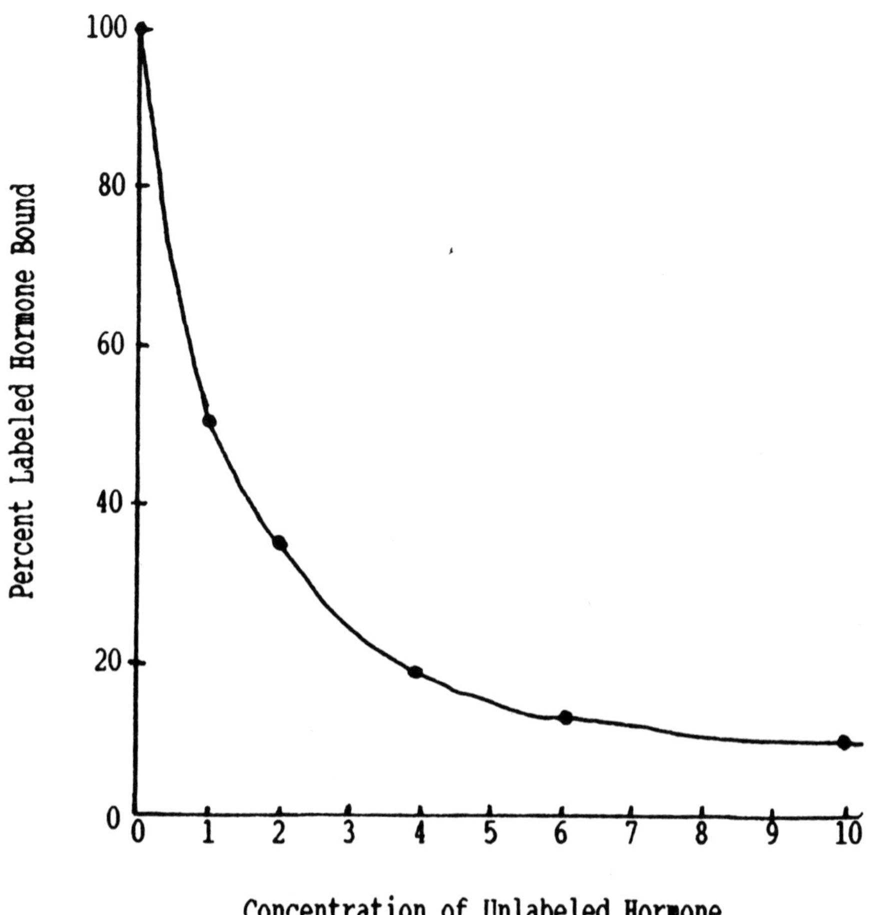

FIGURE 17-4. Binding curve.

ment of the normal distribution of values. It was assumed that hormone values throughout the menstrual cycle would follow a normal distribution so this method was originally used to determine normals. However, in some instances, the arithmetic mean minus two standard deviations gives hormone values that are either zero or negative, a biologic impossibility. It was determined that hormone values follow a log-normal distribution, not a normal distribution. This led to the determinations of the current normal levels. It is still important to use only the values for normal range determined by the laboratory because variability exists among facilities.

Summary

Hormone assays have been greatly improved over the past 30 years. Bioassays are rare in clinical testing. Chemical assays are still used for some hormones, but more often for drug assays. Immunoassays are the most important assays for clinical hormone measurement. Laboratory, in-office tests, and over-the-counter tests (LH, hCG) are available. Their sensitivity and specificity are excellent. It is important to know each laboratory's normal values and the physician should be careful when working with very high or very low values of any given test. If questions arise concerning a reported value, a good laboratory will be able to provide information to the clinician so that correct clinical decisions can be made.

Suggested Reading

Brown JB, MacLeod SC, MacNaughtan C, Smith MA, Smyth B. A rapid method for estimating oestrogens in urine using semi-automatic extractor. J Endocrinol 1968;42:5.

Dufau ML, Mendelson CR, Catt KJ. A highly sensitive in vitro bioassay for luteinizing hormone and chorionic gonadotropin. J Clin Endocrinol 1974;39: 610–613.

Forsyth IA, Myres RP. Human prolactin. Evidence obtained by the bioassay of human plasma. J Endocrinol 1971;51:157–168.

Kletzky OA, Nakamura RM, Thorneycroft IH, et al. Log normal distribution of gonadotropins and ovarian steroid values in the normal menstrual cycle. Am J Obstet Gynecol 1975;121:688.

Klopper A, Michie EA, Brown JB. A method for the determination of urinary pregnandiol. J Endocrinol 1955;12:209–219.

Miles LEM, Hales CM. Labelled antibodies and immunological assay systems. Nature 1968;219:186.

Nakamura RM, Tucker ES, Carlson IH. Immunoassays in the clinical laboratory. In: Henry JB, ed. Clinical diagnosis and management by laboratory methods, 18th ed. Philadelphia: WB Saunders, 1991:848–884.

Roger M, Grenier J, Houlbert C, Castainer M, Feinstein M-C, Scholler R. Rapid radioimmunoassays of plasma LH and estradiol-17β for the prediction of ovulation. J Steroid Biochem 1980;12:403.

Voller A, Bartlett A, Bidwell DE. Immunoassays for the 80's. Baltimore: University Park Press, 1981.

Zondek B, Sulman F, Black R. The hyperemia effect of gonadotropins on the ovary. JAMA 1945;128:939-944.

18.
Amenorrhea

Preston C. Sacks

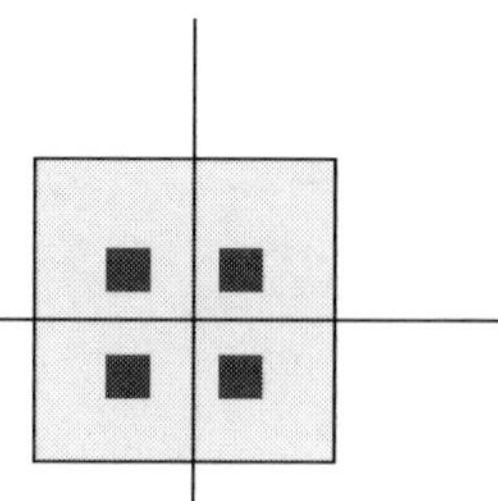

Amenorrhea is defined as the absence of menstrual flow. It is a symptom and not a diagnosis; therefore, the patient presenting with amenorrhea may warrant further evaluation to determine the etiology. Guidelines for pursuing an evaluation are listed in Table 18-1.

Clinical laboratory testing is critical in the evaluation of patients presenting with amenorrhea. An algorithm for laboratory evaluation is presented in Figure 18-1. The remainder of the chapter focuses on the decision steps listed in the algorithm.

Decision I: Is the Patient Pregnant?

Pregnancy can be evaluated by measuring the concentration of human chorionic gonadotropin (hCG) in serum or urine. In early pregnancy, hCG is present in the maternal circulation as the intact molecule (98%), free β subunit (1%), and free α subunit (1%; 1). Intact hCG is the biologically active form; therefore, its assessment is the most critical. Double antibody, two-site "sandwich" immunoassays use antisera, which specifically recognize two sites on the hCG molecule (one on the α subunit and one on the terminal portion of the β subunit).

In vitro studies show that the developing blastocyst begins producing detectable amounts of hCG on day 8 following fertilization (2) and on the day of the missed menses (14 days after fertilization) the level of hCG detectable in the serum of women with normal gestations is roughly 100 mIU/mL (3). Because radioimmunoassays can reliably detect levels of hCG

TABLE 18-1. Guidelines for amenorrhea evaluation

1. No menstruation by age 16

2. No menstruation > 2 ys following initiation of secondary sexual development (ie, thelarche or growth spurt)

3. Amenorrhea has persisted for > 3 mo

4. The clinical situation warrants evaluation (ie, infertility, suspicion of pregnancy, or symptoms and signs to suggest a pathologic cause for amenorrhea)

---

as low as 5 mIU/mL, the diagnosis of pregnancy can easily be confirmed in a sample of serum shortly after the missed menses. One must keep in mind, however, that the hCG levels of women with ectopic gestations or those pregnancies destined for spontaneous abortion may be lower (4).

Recently, nonradiometric assays have gained widespread use in the detection of hCG. These immunoassays are rapid, highly sensitive and eliminate the problems associated with the storage and disposal of radioisotopes. Such assays typically use a chemiluminescent detections system and are so simple to perform and interpret that they have made home and office testing a reasonable alternative to radioimmunoassay.

In our office we use the Abbott TestPack Plus hCG Combo (Abbott Laboratories, Abbott Park, IL). This test kit reliably detects levels of hCG > 25 mIU/mL in a sample of either serum or urine. The results are easy to interpret—a positive sign (+) appears in the result window in < 10 minutes if the sample contains > 25 mIU/mL.

Home pregnancy tests are generally not as sensitive as the in-office tests, with a typical lower limit of detection of 100 mIU/mL. This level is still useful in diagnosing pregnancy as early as the week following the missed menses.

Decision II: Is There an Excess of Prolactin Secretion?

Hyperprolactinemia is present in approximately 20% of patients with secondary amenorrhea (5). The mechanism by which an elevation in serum prolactin leads to amenorrhea is thought to be via inhibition of the pulsatile release of gonadotropin-releasing hormone.

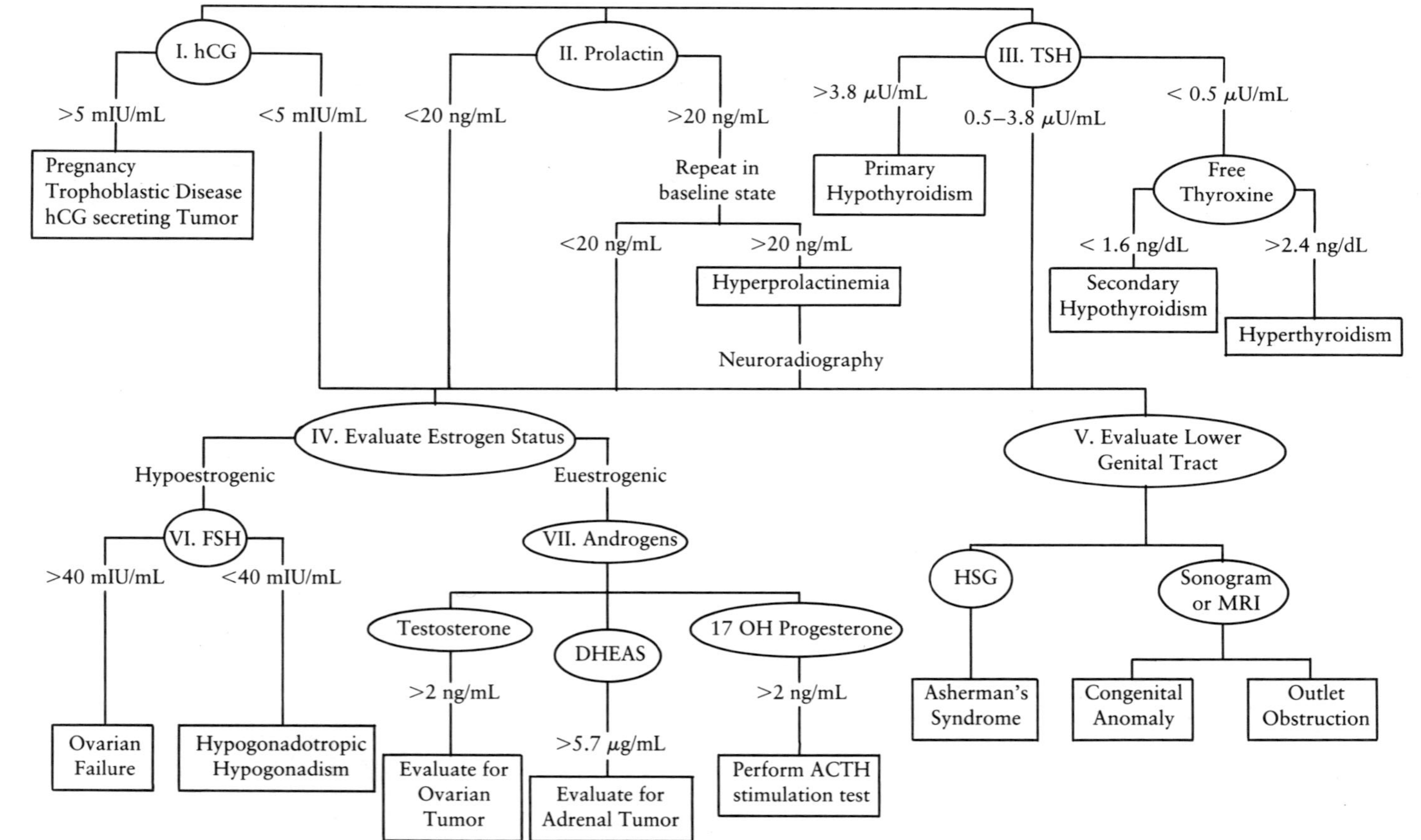

FIGURE 18-1. Laboratory evaluation of amenorrhea

The pattern of prolactin secretion is diurnal, with a peak occurring during nocturnal sleep and a nadir between 9:00 and 11:00 AM. The secretion also varies with the phases of the menstrual cycle (lower in the follicular phase). It is wise to confirm an elevated measurement by repeating the test during optimal baseline conditions (morning sample during the follicular phase). In most laboratories, the upper limit of the normal range for serum prolactin is 20 ng/mL.

Hyperprolactinemia in the absence of an identifiable cause (ie, lactation, pharmacologic agents) is most likely due to a prolactin-secreting pituitary adenoma. Some authors recommend neuroradiologic investigation in all patients with an elevated prolactin level (6). Others recommend investigation only when there is galactorrhea, serum prolactin level > 100 ng/mL, or a finding to suggest an intracranial mass (headache or visual field defects; 7).

Decision III: Is There Dysfunction of the Thyroid Gland?

Hypothyroidism is an important, though uncommon, cause of amenorrhea. Primary hypothyroidism is easily diagnosed by measuring the serum concentration of thyroid-stimulating hormone (TSH). Specific and highly sensitive assays have been developed to accurately measure TSH. The reference range for TSH in most assay systems is 0.50-3.8 μU/mL and any level > 3.8 μU/mL in the absence of other medical illness is virtually diagnostic of primary hypothyroidism.

These ultrasensitive assays also have the added advantage of being accurate when measuring levels < 1.0 μU/mL. This allows for screening of hyperthyroidism, which can also be associated with amenorrhea. TSH levels < 0.5 μU/mL suggest hyperthyroidism or secondary hypothyroidism, and the serum concentration of free thyroxine or calculation of a free thyroxine index (FTI = total $T_4 \times T_3$ resin uptake) should be obtained. The normal range for free thyroxine is 1.6-2.4 ng/dL and the normal range for FTI is 1-4.3 units. Low TSH and thyroxine levels signify secondary hypothyroidism, and the patient should be tested for panhypopituitarism. Low TSH and elevated thyroxine concentrations are found in persons with primary hyperthyroidism and exogenous thyroxine administration.

Decision IV: Is Sufficient Estrogen Present?

This question is usually answered not by the clinical laboratory but rather by a progestin challenge. Any evidence of withdrawal bleeding following progestin administration indicates that sufficient estrogen is present.

Decision V: Is the Lower Genital Tract Normal?

The laboratory plays a role if the uterus is not identified. In its absence, the patient should undergo chromosomal analysis. A female karyotype suggests müllerian agenesis; the finding of a male karyotype is characteristic of androgen insensitivity.

Decision VI: Hypergonadotropic versus Hypogonadotropic Hypoestrogenism?

A decrease in estrogen production may be the result of a primary defect in the ovary or the reduction of gonadotropin secretion from the pituitary gland. The distinction between these two situations is easily made by measuring the serum concentration of follicle-stimulating hormone (FSH). A random serum FSH level of > 40 mIU/mL in an amenorrheic woman signifies ovarian failure.

Once hyperprolactinemia has been excluded, hypoestrogenism in association with low or normal FSH levels is due to hypofunction of the hypothalamus or pituitary gland. This condition is referred to as hypogonadotropic hypogonadism and may result from a multitude of clinical entities including Kallman's syndrome, pituitary failure, eating disorders, simple weight loss, and stress.

Decision VII: Euestrogenic Amenorrhea: PCOS versus CAH and Other Causes of Hyperandrogenism

Amenorrhea in a well-estrogenized woman with a normal endometrium and patent genital outflow tract is due to anovulation. The paradigm of anovulatory amenorrhea is the clinical entity known as polycystic ovarian syndrome (PCOS). In these women androgen production and action are increased. Other clinical conditions, however, may present as PCOS. Congenital adrenal hyperplasia (CAH), Cushing's syndrome, ovarian hyperthecosis, ovarian androgen-producing tumors, and adrenal adenomas may all lead to the clinical picture of polycystic ovaries. The laboratory evaluation is fully discussed in Chapter 20, and more specifics about the ACTH stimulation test are found in Part 7.

References

1. Ozturk M, Bellet D, Manil L, Hennen G, Frydman R, Wands J. Physiological studies of human chorionic gonadotropin (hCG), αhCG, and βhCG as mea-

sured by specific monoclonal immunoradiometric assays. Endocrinology 1987; 120:549–558.

2. Lopata A, Hay DL. The surplus human embryo: its potential for growth, blastulation, hatching, and human chorionic gonadotropin production in culture. Fertil Steril 1989;51:984–991.

3. Lenton EA, Neal LM, Sulaiman R. Plasma concentrations of human chorionic gonadotropin from the time of implantation until the second week of pregnancy. Fertil Steril 1982;37:773–778.

4. Braunstein GD, Karow WG, Gentry WC, Rasor J, Wade ME. First-trimester chorionic gonadotropin measurements as an aid in the diagnosis of early pregnancy disorders. Am J Obstet Gynecol 1978;131:25–32.

5. Franks S, Murray AF, Jequier AM, Steele SJ, Nabarro JDN, Jacobs HS. Incidence and significance of hyperprolactinemia in women with amenorrhea. Clin Endocrinol (Oxf) 1975;4:597–607.

6. Speroff L, Glass RH, Kase NE. eds: Clinical gynecologic endocrinology and infertility, 4th ed. Baltimore: Williams & Wilkins, 1989:165–211.

7. Chang RJ, Keye WR, Young JR, et al. Detection, evaluation, and treatment of pituitary microadenomas in patients with galactorrhea and amenorrhea. Am J Obstet Gynecol 1977;128:356.

Suggested Reading

Azziz R, Zacur HA. 21-Hydroxylase deficiency in female hyperandrogenism: screening and diagnosis. J Clin Endocrinol Metab 1989;69:577–584.

Franks S. Primary and secondary amenorrhea. Br Med J 1987;294:815–819.

Katz E, Adashi EY. Hyperprolactinemic disorders. Clin Obstet Gynecol 1990;33: 622–639.

Klibanski A, Zervas NT. Diagnosis and management of hormone-secreting pituitary adenomas. N Engl J Med 1991;324:822–831.

Latman NS, Bruot BC. Evaluation of home pregnancy test kits. Biomed Instrum Technol 1989;23:144–149.

Thomas R, Reid RL. Thyroid disease and reproductive dysfunction: a review. Obstet Gynecol 1987;70:789–798.

19.
Ovarian Failure

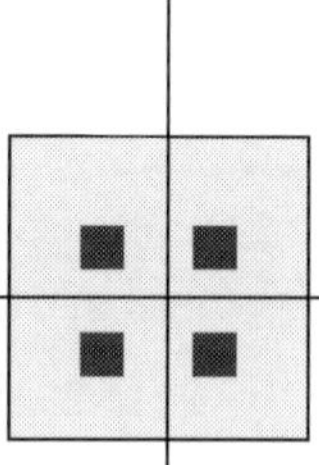

Sanford M. Markham

Ovarian failure may be defined as the lack of, or cessation of, physiologic functions of the ovary, specifically the production of the primary sex hormone, estrogen. Failure of the ovary may occur as a natural event referred to as menopause or at a premature time during the reproductive life due to a variety of etiologies (Table 19-1).

Primary ovarian failure defines women with no previous ovarian function. Secondary ovarian failure defines women who have had ovarian function manifested by the development of secondary sexual characteristics or menses and in whom ovarian function ceases before the time of natural menopause. Premature ovarian failure (POF) has been defined as the cessation of ovarian function at a time prior to natural menopause. A generally accepted age appears to be before age 40 (1). This chapter focuses on the clinical laboratory evaluation of ovarian failure. An overview of the recommended tests is listed in Table 19-2.

Laboratory Diagnosis of Ovarian Failure

Irrespective of the cause, ovarian failure is manifested by an absence of, or a reduction of, estradiol (E_2) produced by the follicular granulosa cells. In primary ovarian failure estrogen-dependent secondary sexual characteristics are either not developed or infantile in size and shape. E_2 and the gonadotropin levels are low. E_2 is generally in the prepubertal range of < 20 pg/mL. Follicle-stimulating hormone (FSH) and luteinizing hormone (LH) values are < 5 mIU/mL. In secondary ovarian failure the E_2 level is also

---

TABLE 19-1. Etiology of premature ovarian failure

1. Autoimmune disorders
2. Cytogenic disorders
3. Enzymatic/hormonal defects
4. Inflammatory disorders
5. Environmental toxins
6. Gonadotropin-resistant ovary syndrome
7. Idiopathic causes

---

typically < 20 pg/mL, but because the hypothalamic-pituitary complex has previously been activated, FSH and LH levels are generally > 40 mIU/mL. In assessing gonadotropins in suspected POF only a FSH level need be drawn. In cases of secondary ovarian failure it is recommended that four separate serum samples for E_2 and FSH be drawn over a one-month period to document the median levels (2).

Laboratory Diagnosis of Autoimmune Disorders Leading to Ovarian Failure

Laboratory testing of the immune system in an evaluation of POF can be divided into three parts: (1) tests of ovarian autoimmune reaction, (2) tests of other organ autoimmune reaction, and (3) tests of systemic autoimmune reaction. These tests are listed in Table 19-3 along with significant results.

The assessment of ovarian autoantibodies has in the past been at best difficult or not available. More recently, increasing numbers of university laboratories and some commercial laboratories have made this test available. Such a test, if positive, would support autoimmunity as a factor in POF; however, it should be noted that a negative test does not totally rule out an autoimmune reaction.

Ovarian autoimmune reaction seldom occurs as an individual event. Multiple systems are often involved with ovarian autoimmune failure. In such cases, the name, "polyglandular failure syndrome," has been applied (3). It is therefore important to evaluate thyroid, adrenal, and parathyroid function. Thyroid tests include T_4, thyroid-stimulating hormone (TSH), thyroid antimicrosomal antibody, and thyroid antithyroglobulin antibody. A finding of reduced circulating T_4 along with an elevated TSH in the presence of thyroid antibodies and ovarian failure would support a diagnosis of polyglandular failure syndrome.

TABLE 19-2. Recommended laboratory evaluation for patients with suspected ovarian failure

A. Tests relating to primary ovarian function (weekly × 4)
 1. Follicle-stimulating hormone
 2. Estradiol
 3. Ovarian biopsy (in selected cases)

B. Tests for cytogenic defects
 1. Chromosomal analysis (karyotype pattern)

C. Tests relating to general endocrine hypofunction
 1. Thyroxine
 2. Thyroid-stimulating hormone
 3. Cortisol (8 AM)
 4. Corticotropin stimulation test
 5. Calcium
 6. Phosphorus

D. Tests relating to metabolic/hematologic dysfunction
 1. Hemogram
 2. Fasting blood sugar/2-h postprandial blood sugar

E. Tests relating to autoimmune defect
 1. Thyroid antimicrosomal antibodies
 2. Thyroid antithyroglobulin antibodies
 3. Anticardiolipin antibody screen
 4. Lupus anticoagulant
 5. Antinuclear antibodies

F. Other endocrine tests
 1. Prolactin

Adrenal assessment may include an 8 AM cortisol level, a corticotropin stimulation test, and antiadrenal antibodies. Polyglandular failure is suggested by a reduced cortisol level followed by a suppressed rise in cortisol in response to corticotropin along with the evidence of ovarian failure.

Hypoparathyroidism has also been seen in cases of ovarian failure. Significant laboratory findings would include reduced serum calcium, elevated

TABLE 19-3. Laboratory testing for autoimmune disorders in ovarian failure

Test	*Significant Result*
Tests of Ovarian Autoimmune Reaction	
1. Antiovarian antibodies	Antibodies detected
2. Ovarian biopsy	Cuff or lymphocytes surrounding follicles
Tests of Other Organ Autoimmune Reaction	
1. Thyroid	
a. Thyroxine	Below lower limits of normal for laboratory assay (nl—4-11 μg/100 mL)[*]
b. Thyroid-stimulating hormone	Above upper limits of normal for laboratory assay (nl—0.6-6 mIU/mL)[*]
c. Thyroid antimicrosomal antibody	Above upper limits of normal for laboratory assay (nl—Titers 1:10)[†]
d. Thyroid antithyroglobulin antibody	Above upper limits of normal for laboratory assay (nl—Titers 1:10)[†]
2. Adrenal	
a. Plasma cortisol (8 AM)	Below lower limits of normal for laboratory assay (nl—5-30 μg/100 mL)[‡]
b. Corticotropin stimulation test	Below lower limits of normal for laboratory procedure (nl—A rise in serum cortisol of > 7 μg/100 mL *or* to a level > 20 μg/100 mL)[‡]
3. Parathyroid	
a. Calcium, serum	Below lower limits of normal for laboratory assay (nl—8.4-10.2 mg/100 mL)[†]
b. Phosphorus, serum	Above upper limits of normal for laboratory assay (nl—2.8-4.5 mg/100 mL)[†]
c. Alkaline phosphatase, serum	Within normal limits for laboratory assay (nl—35-125 IU/mL)[†]
d. Parathyroid hormone (C-terminal)	(nl—0.29-0.85 ng/mL)[§]

Tests of Systemic Autoimmune Reaction

1. Pernicious anemia
   a. Hemoglobin — Below lower limits of normal for laboratory value (12.0–15.0 g/dL)[||]
   b. Hematocrit — for laboratory value (36–46%)[||]

2. Rheumatoid arthritis
   a. Rheumatoid factor titer — >1:40 Titer[||]
   b. Rheumatoid arthritis ' precipitin — Other than negative[¶]

3. Antiphospholipid reaction
   a. Anticardiolipin antibody screen — < 10%[**]
   b. Anticardiolipin IgG antibodies — < 15.0 units/mL[**]
   c. Lupus anticoagulant — Other than negative[**]

4. General autoimmune reaction
   a. Antinuclear antibody — Above upper limits normal for laboratory assay (nl—Titers 0-20)[§]
   b. Total lymphocyte count — Above laboratory normal value (nl—95%)[††]
   c. T cell count — Above laboratory normal value (nl—64-80%)[††]
   d. T_4/T_8 cell ratio — Below laboratory normal value (nl—1.4-2.6)[††]

---

[*]Williams, Textbook of endocrinology, 7th ed. 1985:715, 729
[†]Kohler, Clinical endocrinology, 1986:724, 724
[‡]Yen & Jaffe, Reproductive endocrinology, 2d ed. 1986:712
[§]Maryland Medical Laboratory, Inc., Baltimore, MD
[||]Georgetown University Hospital Laboratory
[¶]Smith Kline Bio-Sciences Laboratory, Lutherville, MD
[**]Diagnostic Assay Services, Gaithersburg, MD
[††]Georgetown University Hospital Immunology Laboratory

serum phosphorus, normal alkaline phosphatase, and decreased parathyroid hormone levels.

Tests of systemic autoimmune reactions include antinuclear antibody (ANA), total lymphocyte count, T cell count, and T_4/T_8 ratio. Patients with autoimmune POF generally exhibit elevated total lymphocyte counts as well as elevated T_4 and T_8 cell counts; however, the T_4/T_8 cell ratio is normally reduced because of the relative larger increase in suppressor-cytotoxic T_8 cells over the helper T_4 cells (4).

Other testing in the evaluation of ovarian failure in polyglandular failure syndrome includes hemogram for pernicious anemia, rheumatoid factor to screen for rheumatoid arthritis, anticardiolipin and lupus anticoagulant to screen for antiphospholipid reaction, and fasting blood sugar and 2-hour postprandial blood sugar to screen for diabetes mellitus.

Laboratory Diagnosis of Cytogenic Disorders Leading to Ovarian Failure

Although the majority of patients with POF have a normal 46,XX karyotype, abnormalities of the X chromosome have been associated with both primary and secondary ovarian failure. The most frequent single cell anomaly is reported to be 45,XO (Turner's syndrome; 5). In addition to an X chromosome monosomy, excess X chromosome defects such as 47,XXX (6), X chromosome structural defects (7), and X autosome translocations (8) may result in POF. Cytogenic studies should initially include a chromosomal assessment using at least 50 lymphocytes from a peripheral blood sample.

Diagnosis of the Gonadotropin-Resistant Ovary Leading to Ovarian Failure

The first reported cases of hypergonadotropic amenorrhea with ovarian failure in the presence of apparently normal ovarian follicles appeared in 1969 (9). Recommended clinical laboratory tests include those discussed previously to rule out ovarian failure and autoimmune disease, prolactin to rule out pituitary tumor, and an ovarian biopsy. Biopsy results reveal a normal complement of primordial follicles with a few antral stage follicles and a variety of atresia stage follicles.

Enzymatic/Hormonal, Inflammatory, and Environmental Causes

The remainder of the etiologies of POF are either rare or require diagnostic modalities using less clinical laboratory assessment. Reported enzymatic/hormonal etiologies for ovarian failure include defects in galactose-1-phosphate uridyl transferase (10) and in 17-hydroxylase (11). Inflammatory conditions leading to ovarian failure include mumps and tuberculosis. Environmental etiologies for ovarian failure include exposure to chemotherapeutic agents and to ionizing radiation.

Summary

The clinical laboratory makes a significant contribution to the diagnosis in the patient presenting with ovarian failure, augmenting the information gained through a careful history and physical examination. Initial diagnosis is assessed through measurement of E_2 and gonadotropins. Tests of systemic immunity and autoimmune disease of other organs are important when evaluating ovarian failure. Chromosomal analysis is also important because of the known relationship between ovarian failure and genetic defects.

References

1. Coulam CB. Premature gonadal failure. Fertil Steril 1982;38:645–655.
2. Rebar RW, Erickson GF, Yen SSC. Idiopathic premature ovarian failure: clinical and endocrine characteristics. Fertil Steril 1982;37:35–41.
3. Coulam CB. Autoimmune ovarian failure. Semin Reprod Endocrinol 1983; 1:161–167.
4. Ho PC, Tang GWK, Fu KH, Fan MC, Lawton JWM. Immunological studies in patients with premature ovarian failure. Obstet Gynecol 1988;71:622–626.
5. McDonough PG, Byrd JR, Tho PT, Mahesh VB. Phenotypic and cytogenetic findings in eighty-two patients with ovarian failure—changing trends. Fertil Steril 1977;28:638–641.
6. Villaneuva AL, Rebar RW. Triple X syndrome and premature ovarian failure. Obstet Gynecol 1983;62(suppl):70S–73S.
7. Coulam CB, Stringfellow S, Hoefnagel D. Evidence for a genetic factor in the etiology of premature ovarian failure. Fertil Steril 1983;40:693–695.
8. Sauer F, Greenstein RM, Reardon P, Riddick DH. Secondary amenorrhea associated with balanced X-autosome translocation. Obstet Gynecol 1977; 49:101–104.
9. Jones GS, deMoraes-Ruehsen M. A new syndrome of amenorrhea in association with hypergonadotropism and apparently normal ovarian follicular apparatus. Am J Obstet Gynecol 1969;104:597–600.
10. Cramer DW, Ravnikar VA, Craighill M, Ng WG, Goldstein DP, Reilly R. Müllerian aplasia associated with maternal deficiency of galactose-1-phosphate uridyl transferase. Fertil Steril 1987;47:930–934.
11. Goldsmith O, Solomon DH, Horton R. Hypogonadism and mineralocorticosteroid excess. N Engl J Med 1967;277:673–677.

20.
Hyperandrogenism

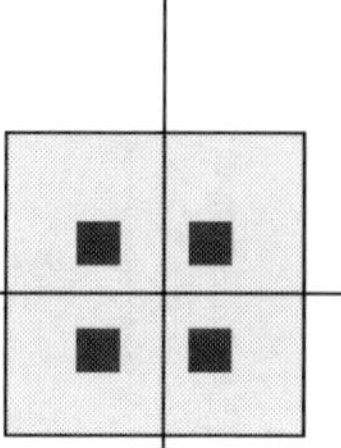

Robert L. Barbieri

Hyperandrogenism is the state of increased androgen production and action. Testosterone and dihydrotestosterone (DHT) are the major androgens in human beings. Androstenedione (AND), dehydroepiandrosterone (DHEA), and dehydroepiandrosterone sulfate (DHEAS) are the major androgen precursors. In most cases of hyperandrogenism the ovary, the adrenal, and the pilosebaceous unit contribute to the androgen overproduction. The primary disorders causing hyperandrogenism are listed in Table 20-1. Androgen overproduction in women is associated with hirsutism, virilization, acne, oligo- or anovulation, infertility, endometrial hyperplasia, and metabolic abnormalities such as hypertriglyceridemia, decreased high-density lipoprotein cholesterol, hypertension, and non–insulin-dependent diabetes mellitus. This chapter reviews the basic clinical laboratory tests that assist the clinician in assessing and managing hyperandrogenism.

Clinical laboratory testing of hyperandrogenic women serves four important purposes: (1) to confirm the history and findings on physical examination, (2) to provide information concerning the severity of the androgen overproduction, (3) to identify the organs involved in the androgen overproduction, and (4) to screen for rare causes of hyperandrogenism.

Table 20-2 lists laboratory tests that may be helpful in evaluating women with hyperandrogenism. The table is divided into two major sets of recommendations. The tests listed as components of the basic testing package are those useful in differentiating among the diseases that can cause hyperandrogenism. The tests listed as components of the optional

TABLE 20-1. Common diseases causing androgen excess

Anovulatory Ovarian Hyperandrogenism (PCOS)	Ovarian Stromal Hyperthecosis	Idiopathic Hirsutism	Adrenal Hyperplasia	Ovarian or Adrenal Tumors	Other (Prolactinoma, Cushing's)
Frequency as a Cause of Hyperandrogenism					
70%	10%	15%	3%	1%	< 1%
Primary Source of Androgen Overproduction					
Ovary, follicles (theca) and stroma	Ovary, stroma	Pilosebaceous unit	Adrenal	Tumor	Adrenal
Secondary Source of Androgen Production					
Adrenal, pilosebaceous unit	Pilosebaceous unit		Ovary, pilosebaceous unit		
Key Features					
Anovulation, hirsutism	Anovulation, hirsutism, virilization may be present	Normal ovulation, hirsutism	Anovulation, hirsutism	Virilization common	
Cause of Disease					
Elevated LH, elevated insulin	Elevated insulin, elevated LH	Overactive 5-α reductase enzyme	Defect 21-hydroxylase enzyme	Genetic mutations	

TABLE 20-2. Laboratory tests useful in evaluating hyperandrogenic women

Anovulatory Ovarian Hyperandrogenism (PCOS)	Ovarian Stromal Hyperthecosis	Idiopathic Hirsutism	Adrenal Hyperplasia	Ovarian or Adrenal Tumors
Basic Test Package				
Total testosterone	Total testosterone	No testing needed	17-Hydroxy-progesterone	Total testosterone
Optional Test Package				
Prolactin, DHEAS, LH, FSH, free testosterone, sex hormone-binding globulin, androstenedione	Glucose tolerance test with measurement of glucose and insulin	$3\alpha{-}5\alpha$-androstanediol glucuronide, androsterone glucuronide, $3\alpha{-}5\alpha$-androstanediol sulfate	Corticotropin stimulation test, deoxycortisol	DHEAS, urinary 17-ketosteroids, androstenedione, sonography of ovaries, magnetic resonance imaging of adrenals and ovaries, selective catheterization of ovarian and adrenal veins

testing package are usually not necessary in the first-line evaluation. Some of these tests are applicable if the patient manifests galactorrhea, virilization, an adnexal mass, or other signs of adrenal disease. Attention is focused in this chapter on the basic testing and a brief description of the role of prolactin, DHEAS, free testosterone, 5 α-reduced steroids, cholesterol, and glucose evaluation in the assessment of these patients.

Total Testosterone

The measurement of total testosterone is a critically important component of the basic laboratory package, and it must be performed by a method with high specificity. Unfortunately, many commercial testosterone assays use antibodies that have significant cross-reactivity with other androgens (such as DHT). In these assays the upper limits to the normal range are often as high as 1.1 ng/mL. In actuality the true range of serum total testosterone in normally cycling women is 0.1-0.75 ng/mL, with a mean of approximately 0.28 ng/mL. Clinicians should review the laboratory they use to ensure that a specific testosterone assay is being used.

If the total testosterone level is 0.7-1.5 ng/mL, ovarian hyperandrogenism is often the cause of the condition. Adrenal hyperplasia due to a 21-hydroxylase defect can also be the cause of a total testosterone in this range, but women with adrenal hyperplasia will have an elevated 17-hydroxyprogesterone level. If the total testosterone value is between 1.5 ng/mL and 2.0 ng/mL, the presence of stromal hyperthecosis should be suspected. If the total testosterone level is > 2 ng/mL, the patient probably has ovarian stromal hyperthecosis or an adrenal or ovarian tumor. If the total testosterone content is < 2 ng/mL in a young woman, an adrenal or ovarian tumor is unlikely to be present.

17-Hydroxyprogesterone

Another key component of the basic test package is the measurement of 17-hydroxyprogesterone. The vast majority of hyperandrogenic women with an elevated 17-hydroxyprogesterone level have 21-hydroxylase deficiency. If the 8 AM 17-hydroxyprogesterone level in the follicular phase of the menstrual cycle is > 4 ng/mL, the patient likely has adrenal hyperplasia due to 21-hydroxylase deficiency. This can be confirmed by a 60-minute corticotropin stimulation test, giving 0.25 mg cosyntropin (ACTH 1-24) intravenously and measuring 17-hydroxyprogesterone 60 minutes later. If the 8 AM 17-hydroxyprogesterone concentration in the follicular phase of the menstrual cycle is < 2 ng/mL, then it is highly unlikely that the patient has adrenal hyperplasia. Women with follicular 8 AM 17-hydroxyprogesterone concentrations between 2 ng/mL and 4 ng/mL probably do not have adrenal hyperplasia, but a corticotropin stimulation test may be necessary to absolutely exclude this possibility. Hyperandrogenic women with adult-onset 21-hydroxylase deficiency are candidates for glucocorticoid treatment and have a definite risk of having children with congenital adrenal hyperplasia.

Dehydroepiandosterone Sulfate

Although DHEAS is largely of adrenal origin, most women with adult-onset adrenal hyperplasia have a normal DHEAS level. In contrast, many women with ovarian hyperandrogenism (polycystic ovarian syndrome [PCOS]) have an elevated DHEAS value. This paradoxical situation limits the utility of the DHEAS measurement in identifying the disease causing the hyperandrogenism. Measurement of DHEAS may have special value in the evaluation of women with hyperandrogenism and infertility. In women with hyperandrogenism, infertility, and a DHEAS level $> 2\mu g/mL$, treatment with dexamethasone may improve the ovarian response to clomiphene and human menopausal gonadotropins. DHEAS measurement may also be of value in evaluating women suspected of having an adrenal tumor. A DHEAS two times greater than the upper limits of normal is consistent with an adrenal carcinoma.

Prolactin

Many authorities recommend that prolactin be measured in all women with anovulation or oligo-ovulation. In a population of anovulatory women without hyperandrogenism approximately 15% of the prolactin measurements will be abnormally elevated. In some reports, as many as 15% of women with anovulatory hyperandrogenism have a mild degree of hyperprolactinemia. However, it is unusual to find a markedly elevated prolactin level in women with anovulatory hyperandrogenism. In a rare woman with anovulatory hyperandrogenism a significantly elevated prolactin concentration is found in association with a prolactin-producing pituitary tumor. In these cases the hyperprolactinemia may be stimulating adrenal androgen production.

Free Testosterone

Most studies of free testosterone demonstrate that it is more sensitive than total testosterone in identifying women with hyperandrogenism.

However, in most laboratories, free testosterone determination is significantly more expensive. It has not yet been demonstrated that the increased expense is justified by the modest increase in sensitivity.

5α-Reduced Steroids

The diagnosis of idiopathic hirsutism can be made on clinical grounds if hirsutism and normal ovulatory cycles are identified. Circulating 5α-reduced steroids (derived from the pilosebaceous unit) are elevated, but measurement of these steroids does not alter clinical care of the patient and therefore is not warranted.

Cholesterol and Diabetic Screening

Many hyperandrogenic women have multiple metabolic abnormalities including insulin resistance, hyperinsulinemia, diabetes, hypertriglyceridemia, hypercholesterolemia, and hypertension. Measurement of total cholesterol and high-density lipoprotein cholesterol and a screen for diabetes may be warranted in hyperandrogenic women.

Suggested Reading

Anderson DC. Sex hormone binding globulin. Clin Endocrinol 1974;3:69.

Azziz R, Zacur HA. 21-Hydroxylase deficiency in female hyperandrogenism: screening and diagnosis. J Clin Endocrinol Metab 1989;69:577-584.

Barbieri RL. Hyperandrogenic disorders. Clin Obstet Gynecol 1990;33:640–654.

Barbieri RL, Smith S, Ryan KJ. The role of hyperinsulinemia in the pathogenesis of ovarian hyperandrogenism. Fertil Steril 1988;50:197–202.

Carlstrom K, Gershagen S, Rannevik G. Free testosterone and testosterone SHBG index in hirsute women: a comparison of diagnostic accuracy. Gynecol Obstet Invest 1987;24:256–261.

Luciano AA, Chapter FK, Sherman BM. Hyperprolactinemia in polycystic ovary syndrome. Fertil Steril 1984;41:719–725.

21.
Hypothalamic Dysfunction in Disorders of Ovarian Cyclicity

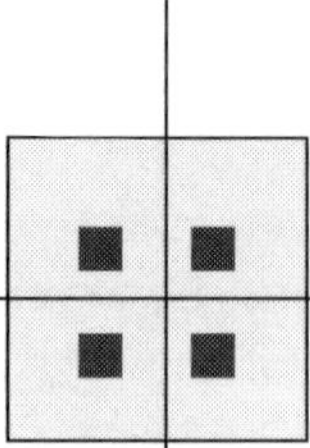

Sarah L. Berga

This chapter focuses on the role of the hypothalamus in disorders of ovarian cyclicity and on the use of the clinical laboratory in the diagnosis of these disorders. Ovarian cyclicity depends on appropriate input from the central nervous system, particularly the hypothalamic gonadotropin-releasing hormone (GnRH) pulse generator. Alterations in the function of the hypothalamus and pituitary either *lead to* or *signal* compromise of gonadal function. It is important to recognize and treat these disorders not only to facilitate conception, but also to protect women from the future development of cardiovascular disease and osteoporosis (1,2).

The GnRH pulse generator refers to a network of GnRH neurons diffusely distributed in the medical basal hypothalamus. This neuronal network has the potential to secrete GnRH in a pulsatile pattern into the portal vasculature and to thereby induce the secretion of the pituitary gonadotropins, luteinizing hormone (LH), and follicle-stimulating hormone (FSH). The GnRH pulse generator is the link between the external environment, the internal milieu, and the ovary. Events or disorders that disrupt the GnRH pulse generator can cause a spectrum of bleeding patterns, including frequent bleeding, short luteal phase with or without shortening of menstrual cycle length, long cycles with or without luteal phases, and complete amenorrhea.

Functional hypothalamic amenorrhea (FHA) is the result of a functional (no organic pathology), and theoretically reversible, slowing of the hypothalamic GnRH pulse generator. LH pulse frequency and mean FSH levels are reduced in women with FHA (3–5), and pulsatile administration of GnRH can restore ovarian cyclicity and result in conception (6,7). Other conditions, however, are associated with either primary or compensatory "hypothalamic dysfunction" and ovarian compromise. These conditions include isolated gonadotropin deficiency, brain tumors, pituitary prolactinomas, other pituitary adenomas, polycystic ovary syndrome, ovarian failure, Cushing's syndrome and disease, and hyper- and hypothyroidism.

The best biochemical evidence in support of the concept that "stress" eventuates in slowing of GnRH release in women with FHA is the consistent demonstration that the activity of the hypothalamic-pituitary-adrenal axis is increased (5,8–10). Exercise, low weight and weight loss, affective and eating disorders, various personality characteristics, drug use, and a variety of external and intrapersonal stresses have been linked to the development of amenorrhea (11,12).

Laboratory Evaluation

After excluding pregnancy, the clinician initially must decide if there is a primary defect at the level of the uterus or vagina such as leiomyomas or Asherman's syndrome versus a disorder that results in ovarian acyclicity. A course of a synthetic progestin can be prescribed to establish that the endometrium is responsive and the outflow tract is patent. In cases of extreme hypoestrogenism, the test may be falsely negative. In this case, a sequential course of estrogen followed by a progestin should be given. The next step is to evaluate the hypothalamic-pituitary-ovarian axis for primary or secondary causes of ovarian acyclicity. An obvious condition to exclude in cases of amenorrhea is ovarian failure. If the ovarian failure is complete, the elevations of LH and FSH will be robust and estradiol levels will be quite low. Because the half-life of FSH is much longer than that of LH, the secretory pattern of FSH in the blood is not pulsatile like that of LH and it is rare for a single blood sample not to detect a significant elevation of FSH. Thus, the clinician can confidently exclude complete ovarian failure by randomly obtaining a single blood sample for FSH and estradiol.

Other common organic disorders that can cause amenorrhea can also be excluded at the same time. If TSH and thyroxine levels are normal, hypothyroidism and hyperthyroidism can be reliably excluded. If the blood sample is obtained between 10:00 AM and noon and before lunch, a normal prolactin level excludes hyperprolactinemia and a pituitary prolactinoma as the cause of amenorrhea.

If the LH, FSH, estradiol, thyroid-stimulating hormone, thyroxine, and prolactin levels are within a normal range, four diagnostic possibilities remain. The two most likely are hyperandrogenic anovulation (HAA) and FHA. The rare possibilities of panhypopituitarism and Cushing's syndrome or disease can generally be excluded by determining free cortisol from a 24-hour collection of urine. A dexamethasone suppression test also may be performed to exclude Cushing's syndrome or disease. If urinary cortisol levels are normal and thyroid axis is intact, panhypopituitarism is unlikely. Because HAA has been associated with hyperinsulinemia and occasionally frank glucose intolerance (13), levels of glucose, insulin, and glycosylated hemoglobin should be assessed.

It may be difficult to convincingly differentiate between mild cases of FHA and HAA. Not all women with hyperandrogenemia are hirsute or have acne. Furthermore, women with FHA may have preexisting hirsutism. Laboratory evaluation is recommended, but it may not reliably discriminate between these two conditions because the circulating levels of LH or any of the androgens other than dehydroepiandrosterone sulfate (DHEAS) are pulsatile. The value of LH of testosterone in a single blood specimen may not be representative of the overall mean level. Because peripheral androgen concentrations may be only marginally increased, the immunoassay performance at low concentrations must be accurate and specific and the normal range in women rigorously ascertained. Estimates of the free component may alleviate this problem in the case of testosterone. Pulsatility can be compensated for by obtaining three to six blood samples at intervals of 10–20 minutes and pooling them (to minimize cost). The reliability of the assessment will then depend primarily on how many samples are obtained. To evaluate the presence or absence of hyperandrogenism, it is recommended that the levels of androstenedione, DHEAS, testosterone, and free testosterone be determined. If the androgen levels are elevated, tumors of the adrenal or ovary, including attenuated forms of congenital adrenal hyperplasia, should be excluded.

If androgen levels are not elevated, the only two possibilities that remain are mild HAA (polycystic ovary syndrome) and FHA. The clinician may seek to corroborate the clinical impression by assessing gonadotropin levels. Because the pituitary function remains intact in both conditions, pituitary stimulation with GnRH does not differentiate reliably between them. Women with HAA may have an acceleration of GnRH and LH pulse frequency and a suppression of FSH secretion, whereas generally women with FHA have a suppression of GnRH and

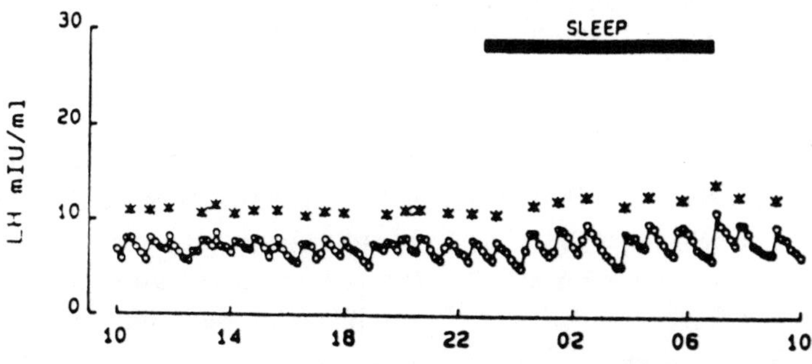
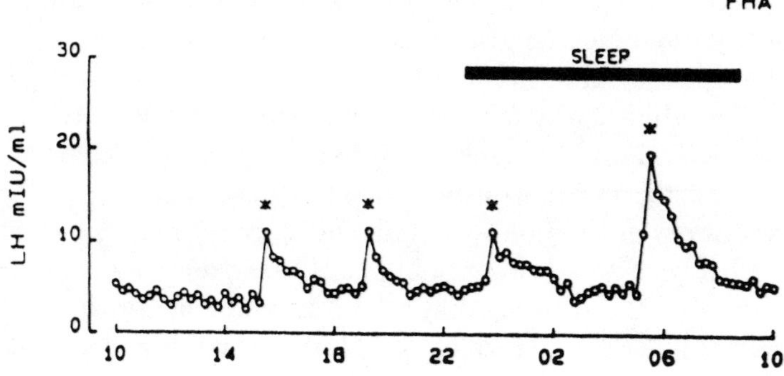
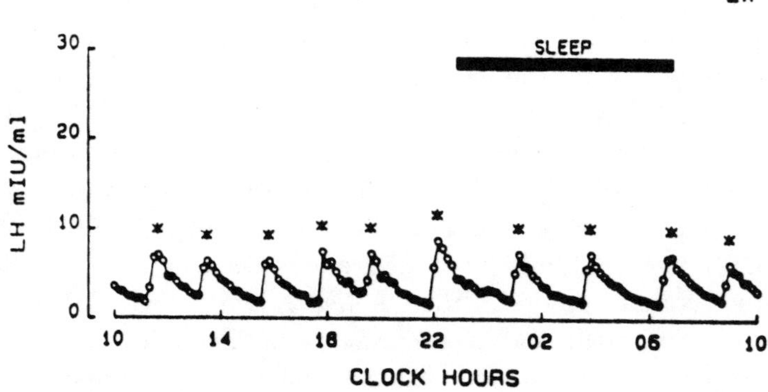

FIGURE 21-1. Representative pulse profiles of LH determined by obtaining blood samples at 15-minute intervals for 24 hours in a woman with hyperandrogenic anovulation or polycystic ovary syndrome (PCO), a woman with functional hypothalamic amenorrhea (FHA), and an eumenorrheic woman (EW) studied in the early follicular phase.

LH pulse frequency and a suppression of FSH. Therefore, logic would predict that the LH/FSH ratio would discriminate between these two conditions. Unfortunately, the pulsatile nature of LH makes it difficult to confidently assess gonadotropin secretory dynamics from a single specimen. Also, newer gonadotropin immunoassays can have different normal ranges and not all are standardized by the same reference preparation. To allow appropriate interpretation of gonadotropin levels, each laboratory must establish the normal range at each menstrual cycle phase for LH, FSH, and the LH/FSH ratio. In a research setting, the LH pulse profile is a "gold standard" for defining the pathophysiology of amenorrheic states. Women with HAA will generally have more than 15 LH pulses/ day, whereas women with FHA will generally have fewer than 10 (Figure 21-1). Although brain tumors are a very rare cause of hypogonadotropic hypogonadism, if there are neurologic symptoms, it is advisable to obtain a magnetic resonance image.

Treatment Implications

Functional hypothalamic oligo- or amenorrhea is largely a diagnosis of exclusion, but it is the only truly reversible cause. A review of the potential life-style variables and mechanisms that contribute to FHA may inspire appropriate life-style alterations and be followed by the "spontaneous" resumption of ovulation. If the FHA appears related to an eating disorder, psychiatric intervention should be considered. Ovulation induction is contraindicated in underweight women (14) or those in whom specific treatment for a concurrent medical condition likely will result in resumption of menses. Regardless of etiology, women with disorders of ovarian cyclicity who are not immediately seeking pregnancy should consider hormonal replacement therapy to guard against the future development of cardiovascular disease and osteoporosis.

References

1. Prior JC, Vigna YV, Schechter MT, Burgess AE. Spinal bone loss and ovulatory disturbances. N Engl J Med 1990;323:1221–1227.
2. Drinkwater BL, Bruemner MS, Chesnut CH III. Menstrual history as a determinant of current bone density in young athletes. JAMA 1990;263:545–548.
3. Reame NE, Sauder SE, Case GD, Kelch RP, Marshall JC. Pulsatile gonadotropin secretion in women with hypothalamic amenorrhea: evidence that reduced frequency of gonadotropin-releasing hormone secretion is the mechanism of persistent anovulation. J Clin Endocrinol Metab 1985;61:851–858.

4. Crowley WF Jr, Filicori M, Spratt DI, Santoro N. The physiology of gonadotropin-releasing hormone (GnRH) secretion in men and women. Recent Prog Horm Res 1985;41:473–526.

5. Berga SL, Mortola JF, Girton B, et al. Neuroendocrine aberrations in women with functional hypothalamic amenorrhea. J Clin Endocrinol Metab 1989; 68:301–308.

6. Hurley DM, Brian R, Outch K, et al. Induction of ovulation and fertility in amenorrheic women by pulsatile low-dose gonadotropin-releasing hormone. N Engl J Med 1984;301:1069–1074.

7. Miller DS, Reid RR, Cetel NS, Rebar RW, Yen SSC. Pulsatile administration of low-dose gonadotropin-releasing hormone: ovulation and pregnancy in women with hypothalamic amenorrhea. JAMA 1983;250:2937–2941.

8. Biller BM, Federoff HJ, Koenig JI, Klibanski A. Abnormal cortisol secretion and responses to corticotropin-releasing hormone in women with hypothalamic amenorrhea. J Clin Endocrinol Metab 1990;70:311–317.

9. Loucks AB, Mortola JF, Girton L, Yen SSC. Alterations in the hypothalamic-pituitary-ovarian and hypothalamic-pituitary-adrenal axes in athletic women. J Clin Endocrinol Metab 1989;68:402–411.

10. Shanan J, Brezinski A, Sulman F, Sharon M. Active coping behavior, anxiety, and cortical steroid excretion in the prediction of transient amenorrhea. Behav Sci 1965;10:461–465.

11. Drew FL. The epidemiology of secondary amenorrhea. J Chronic Dis 1961; 14:396–407.

12. Berga SL, Girton LG. The psychoneuroendocrinology of functional hypothalamic amenorrhea. Psychiatr Clin North Am 1989;12:105–116.

13. Nestler JE, Clore JN, Blackard WG. The central role of obesity (hyperinsulinemia) in the pathogenesis of the polycystic ovary syndrome. Am J Obstet Gynecol 1989;161:1095–1097.

14. Van der Spuy ZM, Steer PJ, McCusker M, Steele SJ, Jacobs HS. Outcome of pregnancy in underweight women after spontaneous and induced ovulation. Br Med J 1988;296:962–965.

Acknowledgments: The technical expertise of Ms. Tammy L. Daniels and secretarial support of Ms. Pat Baeslach are gratefully acknowledged.

22.
Female Fertility

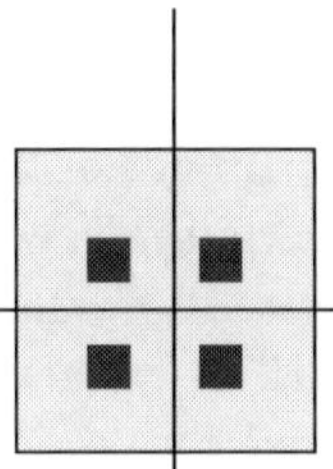

Barry Witten

This chapter provides an overview of the clinical laboratory testing performed on women undergoing fertility evaluation. Additional information regarding some of the tests can also be found in the other endocrine chapters as well as in Part 7.

Hormonal Studies

Follicle-stimulating hormone (FSH) determinations are performed on oligomenorrheic and amenorrheic women. FSH levels > 40 mIU/mL are consistent with women who have developed premature ovarian failure. Basal FSH levels in the range of 20–25 mIU/mL (obtained early in the cycle) are associated with poor ovarian reserve. These patients respond poorly to hyperstimulation regimens and may require donor oocytes.

Basal body temperature (BBT) charting remains an important guide for infertility diagnosis and management. The development of urinary home luteinizing hormone (LH) testing methodologies has augmented BBT monitoring. LH measurement may provide help to couples in timing intercourse and also aid the clinician in the timing of fertility tests. Over-the-counter LH urine tests are available and generally reflect the serum rise in LH, which occurs about 36 hours before ovulation. The test kits have been designed to detect LH levels in the 20–40 mIU/mL range.

Estradiol measurements have been used with FSH in the evaluation of ovarian reserve and also serve (in addition to sonography) to monitor patients undergoing ovulation induction with human menopausal gonadotropin. Basal estradiol values > 50–60 pg/mL are associated with poor ovarian reserve.

Patient history and BBT evaluation are the primary modalities by which the clinician evaluates ovulation. Measurement of progesterone is also occasionally used. Care must be taken with single progesterone determinations because of the pulsatile secretion. A midluteal serum progesterone level of 5–10 ng/mL or greater is indicative of ovulation. Endometrial biopsies are preferred over progesterone determinations for evaluation of luteal phase defect.

Prolactin is measured in oligomenorrheic and amenorrheic women, with or without galactorrhea. Hyperprolactinemia is associated with ovulatory disturbances and luteal phase defect, thus affecting fertility. Thyroid-stimulating hormone should also be measured in women with menstrual cycle disturbances to rule out thyroid disease. Androgen assessment is warranted in patients with menstrual cycle abnormalities and hirsutism. Initial testing includes testosterone, dehydroepiandrosterone sulfate, and 17-hydroxyprogesterone.

Microbiology

Infertility evaluations assess for historical, clinical, and laboratory evidence of inflammation and infection in the genital tract. Cervical testing for *Neisseria gonorrhoeae* and *Chlamydia trachomatis* is performed in addition to evaluation of cervical discharge for cervicitis (numerous leukocytes). Some physicians may attempt to isolate *Mycoplasma hominis* and *Ureaplasma urealyticum* from the cervix. The clinical benefits of searching for these organisms has been debated and many include this as second-line testing. If attempted, the laboratory should be consulted in regard to specimen collection of these fastidious organisms. For patients presenting with chronic pelvic pain or abnormal bleeding, an endometrial aspiration may be performed to test for chlamydia and seek histologic evidence of chronic endometritis.

Postcoital Testing

Although criticized for lack of standardization and interpretation of results, postcoital testing (Sims-Huhner test) remains as a frequently performed test of cervical factor problems. This test of cervical mucus within 2–12 hours following intercourse in used to assess both the quality of the cervical mucus and the presence of motile sperm. Mucus is characterized by amount, stretchability (spinnbarkeit), pH, cellularity, and ferning. Scant mucus may be secondary to prior cervical procedures (eg, cone biopsy). Viscous mucus may be the result of a progesterone effect or drug effect (eg, clomiphene citrate). A question of coital technique may be raised if no sperm are identified. The presence of nonmotile sperm in the cervical mucus may suggest sperm antibodies, acidic pH, or infection. A semen analysis should always be performed in addition to postcoital testing.

Endometrial Biopsy

Endometrial biopsies are obtained in late luteal phase to diagnose luteal phase defects. A phase defect is diagnosed histologically if the secretory pattern shows a lag of > 2 days from what is expected. To ensure an accurate diagnosis, the biopsy needs to be repeated in the following cycle. The appearance of a synchronous versus dysynchronous pattern within the endometrial stroma has been used to guide treatment with either clomiphene citrate or progesterone suppositories.

Suggested Reading

Brodie BL, Wentz AC. Late onset congenital adrenal hyperplasia: a gynecologist perspective. Fertil Steril 1985;48:175–188.

Bronson R, Cooper RG, Rosenfeld D. Sperm antibodies: their role in infertility. Fertil Steril 1984;42:171–183.

Diamond MP. Hyperandrogenism in infertility. J Reprod Med 1989;34:10.

Friberg J. Mycoplasmas and ureaplasmas in infertility and abortion. Fertil Steril 1980;33:351–359.

Gonzalez J, Jezequel F. Influence of the quality of the cervical mucus on sperm penetration: comparison of the morphologic features of spermatozoa in 101 postcoital tests with those in the semen of the husband. Fertil Steril 1985; 44:796–799.

Gump DW, Gibson M, Ashikaga A. Lack of association between genital mycoplasma and infertility. N Engl J Med 1984;310:937–940.

Noyes RW, Hertig A, Rock J. Dating the endometrial biopsy. Fertil Steril 1950;1:3–25.

Scott MG, Landenson JH. Hormonal evaluation of female infertility and reproductive disorders. Clin Chem 1989;35:620–629.

Vermesh M, Kletzky OA, Davajan V, Israel R. Monitoring techniques to predict and detect ovulation. Fertil Steril 1987;47:259–264.

Wentz AC. Endometrial biopsy in the evaluation of infertility. Fertil Steril 1980;33:121–124.

Witten BI, Martin SA. The endometrial biopsy as a guide to the management of luteal phase defect. Fertil Steril 1985;44:460–465.

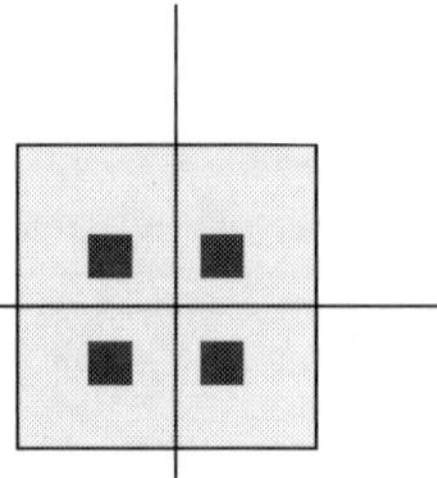

23.
Male Fertility

Michael J. Zinaman
Preston C. Sacks

Infertility affects approximately one in six couples (15%). A male factor can be identified in up to 40% of these cases. Consequently, physicians treating couples for infertility are likely to encounter male factor disorders. This chapter focuses on the clinical laboratory evaluation of the male during the course of an infertility evaluation.

Semen Analysis

The normal parameters of the semen analysis are provided in Table 23-1. If the semen analysis shows a sperm count $> 20 \times 10^6$/cc with a motility of $> 50\%$, a seminal volume > 1.5 ccs, normal sperm morphology of $> 50\%$, and vigorous motility, then little or no further laboratory evaluation is initially warranted. Because variability exists in the results obtained from a single semen test, repeat analysis should be performed if the values are below the aforementioned parameters. If the patient has had exposure to an acute febrile illness or toxin, repeat analysis should be performed in 3 months. This allows for sperm regeneration (the sperm cycle is approximately 72 days).

Ideally, specimens for semen analysis should be collected on site or transported from the patient's home without undue delay at room temperature. Nontoxic specimen containers are required. Abstinence of 48–72 hours before collection helps to avoid problems with decreased ejaculatory volume. Patients with bilateral complete obstruction or congenital absence of the seminal vesicles will not have fructose in the ejaculate in addition to a decreased volume.

TABLE 23-1. Normal parameters on the semen analysis

Volume	> 1.5 cc
Concentration	≥ 20 million/cc
Total sperm count	≥ 40 million
Motility	$> 50\%$
	with 2+ motility or greater
Morphology	$> 50\%$ normal forms
Cellularity	$< 1 \times 10^6$ leukocytes/mL

Sperm motility can assist in predicting male fertility potential. Motility is given both as a percentage of all sperm (normal $\geq 50\%$) and with an indicator of vigor. A subjective numerical grade of 1 to 4 has been used until recently (1). Now computer-aided sperm analysis (CASA) can provide a more objective assessment of motility. If sperm motility is decreased in the presence of a moderate or low sperm count, chronic prostatitis, varicocele, or toxic exposure should be sought. Although there is still some controversy regarding this issue, culture of the seminal plasma for mycoplasma and microscopic evaluation of the seminal fluid for the presence of white cells can be worthwhile (2).

Sperm morphology is a difficult parameter to measure because it requires the subjective views of the technician. Nevertheless the percentage of morphologically normal spermatozoa has been shown to correlate well with the ability to fertilize an ovum (3). In an effort to standardize sperm analysis, Kruger and colleagues have published rigid criteria for the classification of sperm morphology (4). Using their criteria, a normal morphology percentage of $< 14\%$ was associated with a poor rate of fertilization at in vitro fertilization (IVF). This morphologic assessment system is time consuming and has not yet been tested in routine semen analysis to determine whether the predictive ability extends beyond the IVF sphere.

Since the publication of Macomber and Sanders in 1929 (5), sperm concentration has been recognized as an important prediction of male fertility potential. Concentration is generally determined using a hemocytometer. Specialized counting chambers (eg, Makler chamber) are also available and do not require dilution. If the semen analysis demonstrates persistent oligospermia (< 20 million sperm/cc), either with or without decreased sperm motility, it may be worthwhile to assess serum levels of testosterone, luteinizing hormone (LH), and follicle-stimulating hormone

TABLE 23-2. Typical endocrine patterns seen with various causes of male infertility

Condition	Testosterone	LH	FSH
Testicular failure	↓	↑	↑
Hypogonadotropic hypogonadism	↓	↓	↓
Androgen Insensitivity	↑ ↔	↑	↔
Ductal obstruction	↔	↔	↔
Sertoli cell-only syndrome	↔	↔	↑

(FSH). Patients can be classified into various diagnostic categories based on the results of these tests.

Computer-Aided Semen Analysis

As mentioned earlier, computerized analysis can provide a more objective motility evaluation. The normal ranges for these motion parameters are currently under study. Recently, Burkman developed criteria for the identification of hyperactivated sperm using CASA (1). As hyperactivity correlates with sperm capacitation and fertilization potential, it is hoped that CASA will allow for rapid and objective assessment of this important sperm parameter. At this time, CASA has not added significantly to our ability to manage the infertile couple and offers no particular advantage over a well-performed conventional semen analysis.

Endocrine Evaluation

When the initial examination suggests androgen deficiency, or the concentration of sperm is < 20 million/cc, serum testosterone, LH, and FSH concentrations should be determined. Because FSH and LH are secreted in pulsatile fashion, pooling three specimens taken at 15-minute intervals will eliminate an error due to sampling during a pulse peak or nadir. Table 23-2 summarizes the results of these three tests in testicular failure, hypgonadotropic hypogonadism, androgen insensitivity, ductal obstruction, and Sertoli cell-only syndrome.

Additional important points include:

1. Sertoli cell-only syndrome presents with germ cell arrest with normal quantities of Sertoli and Leydig cells.
2. Because fructose is produced in the seminal vesicles, its measurement will help differentiate congenital absence of the vas

deferens and bilateral ductal obstruction from abnormalities in sperm maturation.

3. Prolactin should be measured if pituitary disease is suspected.

Sperm Antibody Testing

When an immunologic cause for infertility is suspected, sperm antibody testing is indicated. The presence of antisperm antibodies may be suggested by significant sperm agglutination on routine semen analysis, shaking sperm on the postcoital test, or failure of fertilization at IVF. Antisperm antibodies are also common in patients following vasectomy and may have prognostic importance in predicting fertility after vasectomy reversal. The presence of antisperm antibodies can be assessed using among others the mixed agglutination reaction or the immunobead test (see Part 7).

Testicular Biopsy

Testicular biopsy is performed on patients with fructose-positive azospermia or severe oligospermia who have normal-sized testes and a normal endocrine profile. If a "wet" preparation shows normal sperm maturation at the time of open biopsy, vasography with duct exploration is warranted.

Assessment of Fertilization Potential

Two tests that have been studied in regard to fertilization potential include the hemizona assay (HZA; 6) and the sperm penetration assay (SPA; 7,8). In the HZA, immature human oocytes with intact zonae pellucida are microbisected into two matched zona hemispheres with qualitatively equal zona surfaces. One hemizona is incubated with the patient's sperm sample, while the matching half is incubated with the sperm of a fertile control. The number of tightly bound sperm is used to calculate an HZA index.

In SPA, mature hamster oocytes are denuded of their zona pellucida to remove the block to cross-species fertilization. These oocytes are then inseminated with a prepared sperm sample from the patient and a fertile control. Results are recorded as the percentage of ova showing sperm binding and penetration (test is considered normal if > 20% of oocytes are penetrated).

References

1. Burkman LJ. Discrimination between nonhyperactivated and classical hyperactivated motility patterns in human spermatozoa using computerized analysis. Fertil Steril 1991;55:363.

2. Styler M, Shapiro SS. Mollicutes (mycoplasma) in infertility. Fertil Steril 1985;44:1–12.
3. Rogers BJ, Bentwood BJ, Van Campen H, Helmbrecht G, Soderdahl D, Hale RW. Sperm morphology assessment as an indicator of human fertilizing capacity. J Androl 1983;4:119–125.
4. Kruger TF, Acosta AA, Simmons KF, Swanson RJ, Matta JF, Oehninger S. Predictive value of abnormal sperm morphology in in vitro fertilization. Fertil Steril 1988;49:112–117.
5. Macomber D, Sanders MB. The spermatozoa count. N Engl J Med 1929;200:981–984.
6. Oehninger S, Coddington CC, Scott R, et al. Hemizona assay: assessment of sperm dysfunction and prediction of in vitro fertilization outcome. Fertil Steril 1989;51:665–670.
7. Yanagimachi R, Yanagimachi H, Rogers BJ. The use of zona-free animal ova as a test system for the assessment of the fertilizing capacity of human spermatozoa. Biol Reprod 1976;15:471.
8. Margalioth EJ, Feinmesser M, Navot D, Mordel N, Bronson RA. The long-term predictive value of the zona-free hamster ova sperm penetration assay. Fertil Steril 1989;52:490–494.

24.
Assisted Reproduction

James P. Toner

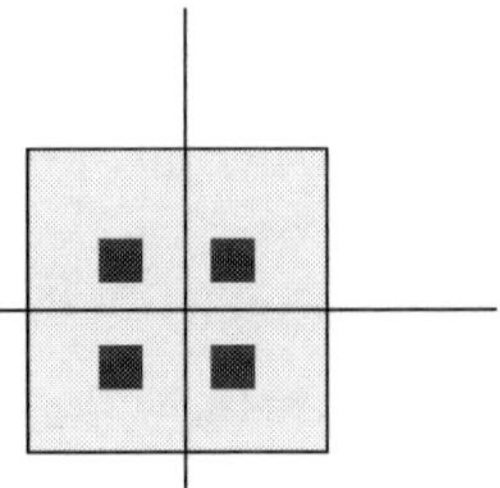

Laboratory testing has been an integral part of successful programs of assisted reproduction from the start. With the arrival of rapid immunoassay methods, several tests have been incorporated into the daily evaluation of patients undergoing ovulation induction. Further, these tests have been used to provide prognostic information about ovarian and testicular reserve, which has been important to clinicians and their patients before embarking on expensive and protracted therapies. This chapter reviews these uses.

Glycoprotein Hormones

Before practitioners apply these tests, it is critical to understand that some commonly used tests (specifically the glycoprotein hormones, follicle-stimulating hormone [FSH], and luteinizing hormone [LH]) give widely different results from laboratory to laboratory and from kit to kit.

Although the amino acid backbones of FSH and LH are generally believed to be invariant, it is clear that these backbones are differentially glycosylated. These different forms exist in different proportions at different times of the cycle. The most potent forms appear to be secreted at midcycle.

Not only are these hormones themselves a *group* of hormones, but the antibodies used to detect them are not equally sensitive to all forms and differ from kit to kit. Because most kit manufacturers were developed independently, most contain unique antibodies not found in other kits.

Practically, this means that one should be careful applying a particular laboratory level cutoff reported in the literature on one's own patients without independent verification of those cutoffs.

Steroid Hormones

Measurements of steroid hormones are subject to less variability than those of glycoprotein hormones. Steroid hormones are invariant in form and show no change in structure in different physiologic conditions. Interlaboratory variability in the measurement of steroid hormones relates to temperature, reagent purity, and inherent noise of radioimmunoassay procedures.

Prediction of Ovarian Response: Use of Basal Hormone Levels

Everyone involved in assisted reproduction has been surprised by the young patient who unexpectedly produces few eggs as well as by women in their forties who produce many eggs. Although this variability in ovarian responsiveness to stimulation has been clear from the beginning, only recently has it been possible to anticipate a particular patient's response with any precision. Given the costs involved and the central role that ovarian responsiveness plays in the success of assisted reproductive technologies, markers of this variability of ovarian reserve are important.

Along with age (1), basal FSH, LH, and estradiol (E_2; 2) levels have proven useful for evaluation of ovarian reserve. Lenton and colleagues (3) have shown that serum levels of FSH in the early follicular phase begin to rise many years before the menopause, as illustrated in Figure 24-1. This rise in FSH can be detected in women contemplating in vitro fertilization (IVF) and can predict performance. This subtle FSH elevation signals declining ovarian reserve even in women with regular menses. Flood and coworkers (4) and Cameron and colleagues (5) among others have reported that some women with unexplained infertility manifest elevations of FSH (although none in the menopausal range), which probably explains their infertility. In IVF, the relationship between FSH and pregnancy rates, as shown in Figure 24-2, is dramatic. As is apparent from data of our clinic (6), pregnancy rates abruptly decline as the basal FSH rises.

Luteinizing hormone and E_2 also show a relationship with IVF performance, but in a less clear cut fashion. Basal LH levels above 25 IU/L are often associated with a polycystic ovarian syndrome-type response in which many eggs of poor quality are produced (2). Basal E_2 levels above 50 pg/mL are also associated with poor response; fewer than half as many

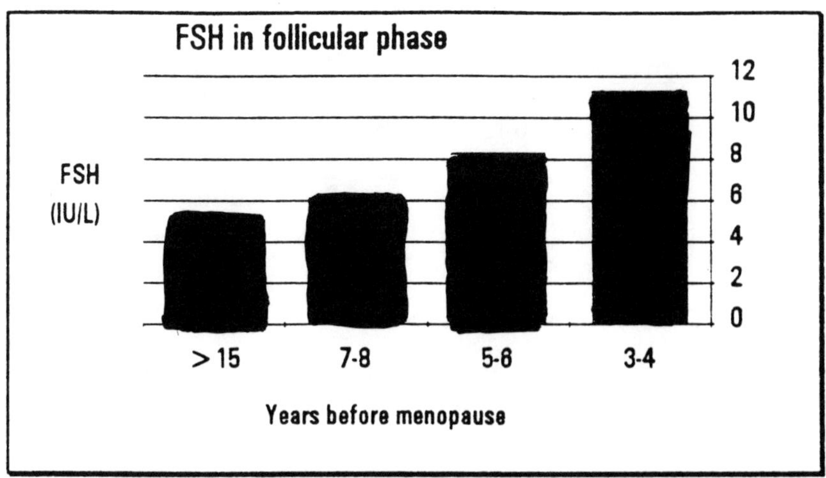

FIGURE 24-1. Basal FSH level rises years before menopause. (Adapted and reproduced by permission from Lenton EA, Sexton L, Lee S, Cooke ID. Progressive changes in LH and FSH and LH:FSH ratio in women throughout reproductive life. Maturitas 1988;10:35.)

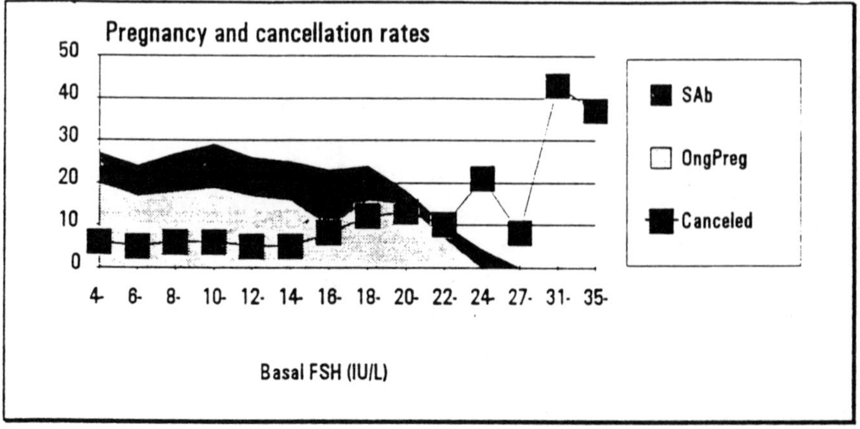

FIGURE 24-2. Relationships between basal FSH and IVF outcomes. (Adapted and reproduced with permission from Toner JP, Philput C, Jones GS, Muasher SJ. Basal follicle stimulating hormone (FSH) level is a better predictor of in vitro fertilization (IVF) performance than age. Fertil Steril 1991;55:784-791.)

pregnancies are observed. This premature E_2 elevation signifies early recruitment and is a common perimenopausal pattern. Interestingly, women with high basal E_2 levels only rarely have a concomitant elevation of their basal FSH, since the inappropriate E_2 elevation effectively suppresses FSH secretion in the menopausal transition.

Levels of FSH have also proven useful in prediction of cryothawed preembryo performance (7) as well as prediction of ovarian reserve in women with one ovary (8).

Provocative Tests of Ovarian Reserve

Dynamic or provocative tests have been studied as predictors of ovarian reserve. In general, they are probably superior to static tests. Their superiority does not come without cost, however. Two recently proposed tests, the clomiphene stimulation test (9,10) and a Lupron challenge test (11,12), although more accurate, take days to complete.

Navot and colleagues (9) used a clomiphene challenge in a group of women over age 35 with unexplained fertility and noted that a high FSH value after the challenge was associated with a low fecundity. Loumaye and colleagues (10) applied this approach to an IVF population by administering 100 mg clomiphene citrate on cycle days 5 through 9. They observed that the sum of FSH measured on day 2 (before clomiphene) and day 10 (after clomiphene) was a better predictor of ovarian response than basal FSH alone. However, the gain in explanatory power was only modest.

Padilla and coworkers (11) have suggested that the E_2 response to early follicular leuprolide acetate administration is predictive of IVF outcome. They administered 0.75–1 mg leuprolide daily beginning on cycle day 2 and saw four patterns of E_2 response. Pregnancy rates associated with these E_2 patterns ranged from 46% when the E_2 level rose abruptly and then fell off to 6% when no E_2 rise could be discerned. We have recently proposed a more succinct provocative test (12) that uses a gonadotropin-releasing hormone agonist given on cycle day 2 (leuprolide acetate 1 mg subcutaneously) with blood assayed on day 2 (before the agonist is administered) and day 3 (24 hours after the agonist). We have observed a strong relationship between the change in E_2 over the one-day period and various measures of IVF success.

References

1. Piette C, deMouzon J, Bachelot A, Spira A. In vitro fertilization: influence of woman's age on pregnancy rates. Hum Reprod 1990;5:56–60.

2. Scott RT, Toner JP, Muasher SJ, Oehninger S, Robinson S, Rosenwaks Z. Follicle-stimulating hormone levels on cycle day 3 are predictive of in vitro fertilization outcome. Fertil Steril 1989;51:651–654.

3. Lenton EA, Sexton L, Lee S, Cooke ID. Progressive changes in LH and FSH and LH:FSH ratio in women throughout reproductive life. Maturitas 1988; 10:35–39.

4. Flood JT, Scott RT, Brzyski RG, Muasher SJ, Denis AL, Jones HW Jr. The occult ovarian factor in unexplained infertility (abstract). Presented at the American College of Obstetricians and Gynecologists Annual Meeting; May 22–25, 1989:22.

5. Cameron IT, O'Shea FC, Rolland JM, Hughes EG, deKretser DM, Healy DL. Occult ovarian failure: A syndrome of infertility, regular menses, and elevated follicle-stimulating hormone concentrations. J Clin Endocrinol Metab 1988; 67:1190–1194.

6. Toner JP, Philput C, Jones GS, Muasher SJ. Basal follicle stimulating hormone (FSH) level is a better predictor of in vitro fertilization (IVF) performance than age. Fertil Steril 1991;55:784–791.

7. Toner JP, Veeck LL, Muasher SJ. Basal FSH and age influence performance of frozen pre-embryos (abstract O-042). Presented at the 47th Annual Meeting of the American Fertility Society, Washington, DC; October 21–24, 1991: S18.

8. Khalifa E, Toner JP, Muasher SJ, Acosta AA. Significance of basal FSH levels in women with one ovary in a program of IVF. Fertil Steril 1992;57:835–839.

9. Navot D, Rosenwaks Z, Margalioth EJ. Prognostic assessment of female fecundity. Lancet 1987;2:645–647.

10. Loumaye E, Billon J-M, Mine J-M, Psalti I, Pensis M, Thomas K. Prediction of individual response to controlled ovarian hyperstimulation by means of a clomiphene citrate challenge test. Fertil Steril 1990;53:295–301.

11. Padilla SL, Bayati J, Garcia JE. Prognostic value of the early serum estradiol response to leuprolide acetate in in-vitro fertilization. Fertil Steril 1990; 53:288–294.

12. Winslow KL, Toner JP, Brzyski RG, Oehninger SC, Acosta AA, Muasher SJ. The gonadotropin-releasing hormone agonist stimulation test—a sensitive predictor of performance in the flare-up in vitro fertilization cycle. Fertil Steril 1991;56:711–717.

25.
Oral Contraceptives

George T. Koulianos
Ian H. Thorneycroft

Oral contraceptives (OCs) have been used in clinical practice since 1960. The first contraceptive commercially marketed contained 0.150 mg mestranol and 9.85 mg norethynodrel (Enovid). Since then, these medications have undergone a great deal of study and modification to maintain their effectiveness while diminishing their side effects. Lower dosages, alteration of dosage during the cycle, and the recent introduction of new progestins are the major modifications that have occurred with OCs since their inception. This chapter focuses on laboratory test alterations (Table 25-1) that occur as a side effect of pill usage.

Gonadotropin-Releasing Hormone Suppression

Oral contraceptives prevent the midcycle gonadotropin surge and ovulation primarily by suppressing the release of gonadotropin-releasing hormone (GnRH) from the hypothalamus (1). OCs also exert a direct effect on the pituitary with suppression of follicle-stimulating hormone (FSH) and luteinizing hormone (LH). FSH and LH levels in women on OCs tend to be low. Once the woman discontinues OCs, the interval needed for gonadotropin levels to return to normal is variable. In most patients FSH and LH will return to normal within 4 weeks.

Alteration in Binding Proteins

Binding proteins produced by the liver include sex hormone-binding globulin (SHBG), cortisol-binding globulin (CBG), and thyroid-binding globulin (TBG). Binding proteins are important because only free fractions

TABLE 25-1. Oral contraceptive and laboratory testing alteration

Gonadotropin-releasing hormone suppression
Alteration in binding proteins
    Sex hormone-binding protein
    Cortisol-binding globulin
    Thyroid-binding globulin
    Hematologic alterations secondary to reduced
    menstrual flow
Coagulation alterations
Alteration of carbohydrate metabolism
Lipid alterations

of steroid hormones are biologically active while bound fractions are inactive. These proteins are elevated in patients taking OCs secondary to the estrogen component.

The principal binding protein for androgens is SHBG, and 80% to 85% of testosterone is bound to SHBG. Pharmacologic agents such as OCs that increase SHBG will also increase the bound fraction of androgens and decrease the free or biologically active fraction. This is especially important in hyperandrogenic conditions such as polycystic ovarian syndrome and hirsutism. By using OCs, one can decrease free testosterone levels and thus help minimize the hyperandrogenic sequelae of this condition. Table 25-2 reviews SHBG and testosterone changes observed with various OCs. In general, although some variability is noted between OC formulations, the net clinical effect is the same.

Transcortin or CBG is the principal binding globulin for cortisol and progesterone. Approximately 75% of cortisol and 10% of progesterone is CBG bound. There is little or no sex difference in plasma CBG levels. The effect of OCs on plasma cortisol and CBG levels is not as thoroughly understood as the effect of OCs on androgens and SHBG. The estrogen fraction of OCs mildly elevates CBG and total cortisol levels while free levels are unchanged (2). Cortisol levels would be in the normal to high normal range.

Oral contraceptives affect thyroid function tests by enhancing carrier protein synthesis in the liver. The estrogen portion of OCs increase TBG synthesis by the liver. This results in increases in total T_4, total T_3, and reverse total T_3 while T_3 resin uptake declines. Free T_4 and free T_3 are not

TABLE 25-2. Effect of oral contraceptives on SHBG, total and free testosterone (T) in normal women

	(% change)		
Oral Contraceptive	*SHBG*	*Total T*	*Free T*
EE 30, 40, 30 μg			
LG 0.05, 0.075, 0.125 mg	92	-26	-35
(Triphasil)			
EE 30 μg; NG 0.3 mg (Lo-Ovral)	24	-21	-37
EE 35 μg; NE 0.4 mg (Ovcon)	271	-3	-49
EE 35 μg; NE 1.0 mg	92	-36	—
(Ortho Novum 1/35)			
EE 30 μg; LG 0.15 mg (Nordette)	28	-16	-31

EE, ethinyl estradiol; LG, levonorgestrel; NG, norgestrel; NE, norethindrone; — not reported

Reprinted from: Koulianos GT, Thorneycroft IH. Abnormal sex hormone binding globulin. In: Schlaff WD, Rock JA, eds. Decision making in reproductive endocrinology. Boston: Blackwell Scientific Publications, 1993, pg. 244

affected. Although total T_4 is mildly elevated, these patients are clinically euthyroid because free T_4 is unchanged. When evaluating thyroid status in women, one should ask if the patient is taking OCs. When evaluating thyroid status in OC users, the clinician should use free T_4 and thyroid-stimulating hormone (TSH) because increases in TBG can affect other tests. Table 25-3 illustrates the effect of OCs on thyroid function tests.

Hematologic Alterations Secondary to Menstrual Flow Reduction

One of the principal benefits of OCs is that they reduce menstrual flow. A number of investigators have confirmed that women on OCs lose one third to one half the menstrual blood iron when compared to women not on OCs. Thein and colleagues noted that the median menstrual iron loss for women not on OCs was 0.51 mg/day compared to 0.15 mg/day for OC users (3). Nilson and Slovell found that menstrual blood loss before using OCs was on average 30.8 ± 14.3 mL and decreased to 14.2 ± 0.9 mL with OC use (4). Further confirmation that women on OCs bleed less comes from the Royal College of General Practitioners who reported that the rate of diagnosed iron deficiency anemia among 23,606 women taking OCs was only 0.56 times the rate for women who had never used OCs (5).

TABLE 25-3. Effect of oral contraceptives on thyroid function

Parameter	Control	OC User	P
Total T_4 (ng/mL)	71.2±9.3	107.5±20.4	<0.01
Total T_3 (ng/mL)	114.5±22.5	162.8±33.9	<0.01
Free T_4 (pg/mL)	12.3±1.35	11.5±1.3	NS
Free T_3 (pg/mL)	4.3±0.4	4.0±0.3	NS
Reverse T_3 (ng/100 mL)	19.6±3.25	27.3±4.0	<0.01
Free T_4 index (units)	2.5±0.2	3.0±0.7	<0.01
T_3 resin uptake (%)	28.9±1.6	25.3±1.7	NS
TBG (μg/mL)	16.1±2.3	34.4±10.0	<0.01

Adapted from: Pansini F, et al. Effect of hormonal contraception on serum reverse triiodothyroxine levels. Gynecol Obstet Invest 1987;23:133–134. Swanson MA, et al. Free thyroxine and free thyroxine index in women taking oral contraceptives. Clin Nucl Med 1981;4:168–171.

Frassinelli-Gunderson and coworkers compared complete blood counts and iron stores in 71 women not on OCs with 46 women who have been on OCs for at least 3 years (6). Their findings are summarized in Table 25-4. The increase in iron stores as demonstrated by a 50% increase in serum ferritin in the OC users is probably secondary to either diminished menstrual blood loss or estrogenic stimulation of apoferritin synthesis by the liver. The decline in erythrocyte volume and lack of an increase in hemoglobin and hematocrit are due to an estrogen-related increase in plasma volume. Walters and Lim demonstrated an increase in plasma volume from 3.138 ± 0.333 L before OC use to 3.488 ± 0.452 L with OC use (7). This dilutional effect causes erythrocyte volume to decline. The higher mean corpuscular hemoglobin concentration and mean corpuscular hemoglobin reflect improved iron status at the cellular level. Increases in serum transferrin, total iron-binding capacity, and serum iron reflect estrogenic stimulation of liver proteins.

Alteration in Coagulation

Mead examined factor VII and fibrinogen levels in women using 30 μg and 50 μg formulations and demonstrated a dose-dependent increase in both factors (8; Table 25-5). It is important to note that the increased risk of thromboembolic phenomenon has primarily been demonstrated in women using only high-dose formulations ($\geq$ 50 μg ethinyl estradiol).

TABLE 25-4. Effect of oral contraceptives on Complete Blood Count and iron stores

Parameter	Control	OC User	P
RBC × 103	4.5±0.26	4.33±0.29	<0.001
Hemoglobin (g %)	13.4±0.98	13.3 ±0.68	NS
Hematocrit (volume %)	39.4±2.4	38.4 ±1.9	<0.05
MCV (μ^3)	87.4±3.96	88.8 ±3.92	NS
MCH ($\mu\mu$g)	29.9±1.8	30.8 ±1.4	<0.01
MCHC (%)	33.5±1.2	33.98±0.66	<0.015
Serum ferritin (ng/mL)	25.4±15.96	39.5 ±21.5	<0.001
Serum transferrin (mg/dL)	266.1±43.3	301.7 ±35.9	<0.001
Serum iron (μg/dL)	104.0±34.3	132.7 ±47.6	<0.001
TIBC (μg/dL)	373.6±44.8	425.4 ±43.0	<0.001

Adapted from: Frassinelli-Gunderson EP, et al. Iron stores in users of oral contraceptive agents. Am J Clin Nutr 1985;41:703–712.

MCH, mean corpuscular hemoglobin; MCHC, mean corpuscular hemoglobin concentration; MCV, mean corpuscular volume; RBC, red blood cell count; TIBC, total iron-binding capacity

TABLE 25-5. Age-adjusted factor VII and fibrinogen levels by oral contraceptive dose

		Estrogen dose	
	Not on OCs	30 μg	50 μg
Number of patients	243.0	15.0	65.0
Factor VII (%)	83.0	96.6	121.1
Fibrinogen (g/L)	2.52	2.84	2.89

Adapted from: Mead TW. Oral contraceptives, clotting factors, and thrombosis. Am J Obstet Gynecol 1982;142:758–761.

Alteration in Carbohydrate Metabolism

The progestin component of OCs exerts a mild dose-dependent effect on carbohydrate metabolism. This effect is especially evident in high-dose formulations. In a national survey the average incidence of glucose intolerance was 15.4% in OC users compared to 6.3% in nonusers (9). OC use increased one- and two-hour plasma glucose levels by 14 mg/dL and 13 mg/dL, respectively. This effect is reversible with discontinuation of OCs. Unfortunately, this study was done with higher dose formulations than currently available. With currently available low-dose formulations OC users undergoing glucose tolerance testing demonstrate only mild and clinically insignificant impairment of glucose tolerance (10).

Alteration in Lipid Metabolism

Estrogens and progestins exert opposite effects on lipid metabolism. Estrogens exert a dose-dependent effect, raising high-density lipoprotein (HDL), lowering low-density lipoprotein (LDL), and increasing total cholesterol and triglyceride levels. Progestins exert an opposite dose-dependent effect, tending to lower HDL and total cholesterol while raising LDL. Progestins do not affect triglycerides. Although different progestins in OCs have different potencies, the doses used in OCs are adjusted such that they all exert similar effects on lipids. The lipid changes exerted by low-dose OCs do not appear to be clinically significant. Also there appears to be little if any difference between various low-dose OC formulations.

The New Progestins

New oral contraceptives containing the progestogens desogestrel, norgestimate, and gestodene have been introduced in the United States (11–13). These progestogens have minimal androgenic side effects. These formulations appear to show similar or even lesser impact on carbohydrate and lipid metabolism compared to other preparations.

References

1. Mishell DR. Oral steroid contraceptives. In: Mishell DR, ed. Infertility, contraception, and reproductive endocrinology. Boston: Blackwell Scientific, 1991:839.
2. Yen SSC. Chronic anovulation caused by peripheral endocrine disorders. In: Yen SSC, Jaffe RB, eds. Reproductive endocrinology. Philadelphia: WB Saunders, 1986:441–476.
3. Thein M, Beaton GH, Milne H. Oral contraceptive drugs: some observations on their effect on menstrual loss and hematological indices. Can Med Assoc J 1969;101:73.
4. Nilson L, Slovell L. Clinical studies on oral contraceptives—a randomized double blind, crossover study of 4 different preparations (Anovlar mite, Lyndiol mite, Ovulen and Volidan). Acta Obstet Gynaec Scand 1967;46(suppl 8):1–31.

5. Royal College of General Practitioners. Oral contraceptives and health: an interim report from the oral contraception study of the Royal College of General Practitioners. London: Pitman Medical, 1974.

6. Frassinelli–Gunderson EP, Margen S, Brown JR. Iron stores in users of oral contraceptive agents. Am J Clin Nutr 1985;41:703–712.

7. Walters WAW, Lim YL. Haemodynamic changes in women taking oral contraceptives. J Obstet Gynaec Br Cwlth 1970;77:1007–1012.

8. Mead TW: Oral contraceptives, clotting factors, and thrombosis. Am J Obstet Gynecol 1982;142:758–761.

9. Russell R, Ezzati TM, Perlman JA, et al. Impaired glucose tolerance in women using oral contraceptives: United States, 1976–1980. J Chron Dis 1987; 40:3–11.

10. Gillespy MJ, Notelovitz M, Ellingson AB, Khan FY. Effect of long term triphasic oral contraceptive use on glucose tolerance and insulin secretion. Obstet Gynecol 1991;78:108–110.

11. Godsland IF, Crook D, Simpson R, et al. The effects of different formulations of oral contraceptive agents on lipid and carbohydrate metabolism. N Engl J Med 1990;323:1375–1381.

12. London RS, Chapdelaine A, Upmalis D, Olson W, Smith J. Comparative contraceptive efficacy and mechanism of action of the norgestimate-containing triphasic oral contraceptive. Acta Obstet Gynecol Scand Suppl 1992;156:9–14.

13. London RS. The new era in oral contraception: pills containing gestodene, norgestimate, and desogestrel. Obstet Gynecol Surv 1992;47:777–782.

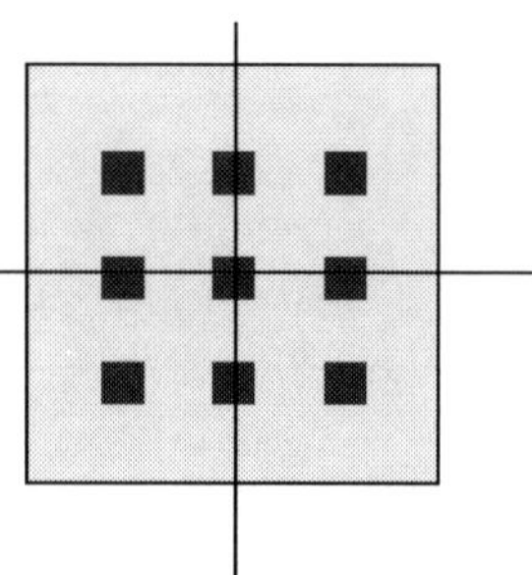

PART SIX
Gynecologic Oncology

26.
Tumor Markers

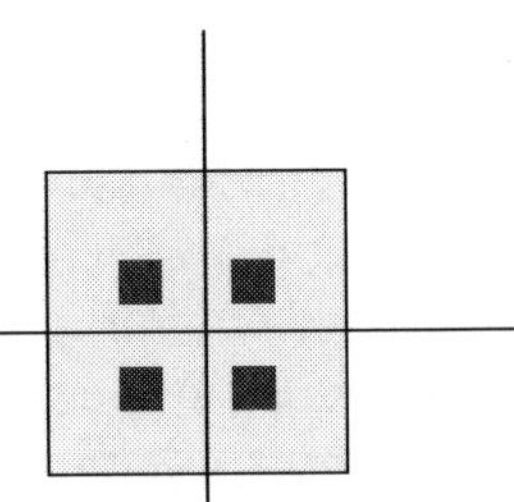

Ronald K. Potkul

The use of the tumor marker depends on the liberation of such substances in the blood or other bodily fluids in concentrations not usually found in the normal population. The substances can be hormones such as human chorionic gonadotropin (hCG), tumor-associated antigens such as the CA125 or oncofetal antigens such as α-fetoprotein (AFP, produced by germ cell tumors containing yolk sac elements and hepatocellular carcinomas), and carcinoembryonic antigen (produced by tumors of the gastrointestinal tract).

CA125

CA125 is an antigenic determinate expressed by more than 80% of nonmucinous ovarian adenocarcinomas (1). The antigen can be measured in serum using radioimmunoassays with a positive level defined as > 35 units/mL in most laboratories. Although > 80% of patients with an ovarian adenocarcinoma will have an elevated CA125 (> 35 units/mL), it can also be elevated in patients without ovarian malignancies (1,2). Among healthy blood donors, the CA125 level was > 35 units/mL in 1% of women. Elevations in the CA125 have also been observed in a variety of benign conditions including pregnancy, endometriosis, pelvic inflammatory disease, adenomyosis, pancreatitis, chronic alcoholic hepatitis, and renal failure. So an elevated CA125 level of > 35 units/mL does not definitively imply that the patient has ovarian cancer.

The CA125 assay can be helpful in monitoring patients with ovarian cancer (1). If initially elevated, the levels correlate well with the patient's disease course. Persistently rising values of CA125 have been consistently associated with progressive disease. In contrast, falling levels imply a clinical response to therapy. Unfortunately, return to negative values does not guarantee a complete response because patients who undergo restaging laparotomies are found to have persistent disease in about one half the cases with negative preoperative CA125 levels (3).

CA125 has also been useful in distinguishing benign from malignant pelvic masses. One study by Patsner and Mann evaluated 250 consecutive patients with pelvic masses who underwent surgical evaluation (4). Seventy-two percent of patients subsequently found to have ovarian cancer had an elevated CA125 and only 20% of patients with negative CA125 had malignant disease, giving a positive predictive value of 0.79. This implies that a patient with an elevated CA125 and a pelvic mass has a 79% chance of having an ovarian malignancy. On the surface these results are encouraging although looking solely at patients with stage I disease, only 4 of 14 cases demonstrated an elevated CA125 (sensitivity = 0.28). This is disheartening because these are the specific ovarian cancer patients we would like to detect early.

CA125 is not useful as a screening test in patients without adnexal masses. A study from Stockholm has screened 5550 women with annual serum assays (5). Among 175 women with an elevated CA125 level, 6 ovarian cancers were detected. The positive predictive value of the CA125 was only 3.4% and 4 of these patients (67%) had disease that had spread outside of the ovary at diagnosis. A second study tested 1010 post-menopausal volunteers (6). One case of ovarian cancer was detected by screening with a CA125 level equal to 32 units/mL. None of the remainder of the patients presented with ovarian cancer after 2 years of follow-up. With the use of 30 units/mL as a cutoff, the sensitivity was 100%, the specificity was .97 (false positive rate was 3%), and the odds of having ovarian cancer given a positive result were only 1 of 300 patients with a CA125 level >30 units/mL. These low positive predictive values (< 0.04) question the routine application of CA125 as a screening tool for ovarian cancer in the general population.

α-Fetoprotein

α-Fetoprotein is a glycoprotein produced by fetal tissue of the yolk sac, liver, and upper gastrointestinal tract (7). After birth, AFP disappears rapidly from the serum and 3 weeks after full-term delivery it only can be detected in small amounts ($<$ 15 ng/mL). Elevated serum AFP levels in nonpregnant patients are found in hepatocellular carcinoma, germ cell tumors with yolk sac differentiation (endodermal sinus and embryonal tumors), and occasionally in cancers of the pancreas, stomach, or biliary system. It is a very specific marker in germ cell tumors of the ovary. This has become increasingly important in follow-up as chemotherapy for germ cell tumors with endodermal sinus elements has become more effective. Pure dysgerminomas, which often require no additional therapy for stage I, can have a mild elevation of human chorionic gonadotropin (hCG; $<$100 mU/mL), but any elevation in AFP implies a mixed tumor containing some yolk sac elements that require aggressive adjuvant chemotherapy (8). It is important to always obtain the serum tumor markers when germ cell tumors are expected preoperatively or if found at the time of surgery.

Human Chorionic Gonadotropin

Human chorionic gonadotropin is a glycoprotein hormone produced by trophoblastic cells of the placenta or syncytiotrophoblast-like cells of gestational trophoblastic disease or germ cell tumors. The quantitative β-hCG assay is as close to an ideal tumor marker that is available in medicine today. In the case of gestational trophoblastic disease, we treat a positive tumor marker itself no longer requiring pathologic confirmation for diagnosis. It is also exceptional in evaluating tumor response. No longer must we wait for gross tumor enlargement to determine chemotherapy resistance before selecting an alternate chemotherapeutic agent. The β-hCG assay is discussed in greater detail in Chapter 28. β-hCG can also be an acceptable marker in germ cell tumors of the ovary such as nongestational choriocarcinoma and embryonal tumors. The β-hCG assay may be mildly elevated in a pure dysgerminoma, which contains isolated gonadotropin-producing syncytiotrophoblastic giant cells (9). If the hCG level is $>$ 100 mU/mL, a diagnosis of a mixed germ cell tumor must be considered and the patient treated aggressively.

Lactic Acid Dehydrogenase

Serum lactic acid dehydrogenase (LDH) is also a potentially useful marker in dysgerminomas (10). The LDH level tends to be higher in dysgerminomas as compared to epithelial ovarian cancer. Interestingly, the elevated fractions of LDH are reversed between dysgerminomas and epithelial ovarian cancer. In epithelial cancers LDH-3, LDH-4, and LDH-5 are elevated in contrast to the higher LDH-1 and LDH-2 fractions found in dysgerminomas.

Hormone Receptors

It is now generally accepted that the interaction of a steroid hormone with an intracellular receptor protein is the primary event that triggers a specific hormonal response in the target tissue such as breast and endometrium. These receptors can be measured and this measurement can assist the clinician in the choice of appropriate treatment. Breast cancers that are estrogen and progesterone receptor positive are more likely to respond to hormonal therapy (11), whereas those tumors lacking receptors are less likely to benefit from progesterone or tamoxifen.

The relationship for hormonal receptors and endometrial cancer is less clear. Although it has been known for some time that about a third of patients with advanced or recurrent endometrial cancer will respond to progestational therapy, no accurate test distinguishes this group from the progesterone nonresponders. Although these problems make the determination of estrogen and progesterone receptors in gynecologic malignancy less than optimal, they are not without benefit. Tissues from an endometrial cancer and a recurrent ovarian cancer should be submitted for hormonal receptor status because chemotherapy in these instances is often less than optimal, suggesting that these patients would probably benefit from a trial of hormonal manipulations since the treatment-related toxicities are so minimal.

References

1. Bast RC, Clug TL, St. John E, et al. A radioimmunoassay using a monoclonal antibody to monitor the course of epithelial ovarian carcinoma. N Engl J Med 1983;309:169–171.
2. Jacobs IJ, Bast RC. The CA125 tumor associated antigen; a review of the literature. Hum Reprod 1989;4:1–12.
3. Berek JS, Knapp RC, Malkasian GD, et al. CA125 serum levels correlated with second-look operations among ovarian cancer patients. Obstet Gynecol 1986;67:685–689.
4. Patsner B, Mann WJ. The value of pre-operative serum CA125 levels in patients with pelvic mass. Am J Obstet Gynecol 1988;159:873–876.
5. Einhorn N, Sjoval K, Schoenfeld G, et al. Early detection of ovarian cancer using the CA125 radioimmunoassay. Am Soc Clin Oncol 1990;9:157–161.
6. Jacobs IJ, Stabile I, Bridges J, et al. Multinodal approach to screening for ovarian cancer. Lancet 1988;1:263–271.

7. Gitlin D, Pericelli A, Gitlin G. Synthesis of alpha-fetoprotein by liver, yolk sac and gastrointestinal tract of the human conceptus. Cancer Res 1972;32:979–982.

8. Talerman A, Haije WG, Baggerman L. Serum alpha-fetoprotein (AFP) in patients with germ cell tumors of the gonads and extragonadal sites. Correlation between endodermal sinus (yolk sac) tumor and raised serum AFP. Cancer 1980;46:380–385.

9. Knapp DS, Kohorn EI, Merino MJ, Livolsi VA. Pure dysgerminoma of the ovary with elevated serum human chorionic gonadotropin: Diagnostic and therapeutic considerations. Gynecol Oncol 1985;20:234–244.

10. Fujii S, Konishi I, Suzuki A, et al. Analysis of serum lactic dehydrogenase levels and its isoenzymes in ovarian dysgerminoma. Gynecol Oncol 1985;22:65–72.

11. McGuire WL. Hormones, receptors and breast cancer. New York: Raven Press 1978.

27.
Laboratory Alterations Encountered in Managing Gynecologic Malignancies

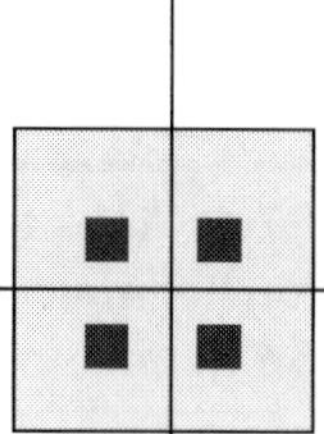

George Lewandowski
Larry J. Copeland

This chapter focuses on the use of clinical laboratory tests in gynecologic oncology patients. In particular, the laboratory alterations seen with radiation and chemotherapy, renal and hepatic complications, nutritional disturbances, and paraneoplastic syndromes are highlighted.

Bone Marrow Suppression

Antineoplastic treatments such as chemotherapy and radiation therapy commonly result in both acute and chronic bone marrow suppression. Patterns of depression of white blood cells (WBCs), red blood cells (RBCs), and platelets can often be predicted based on the particular chemotherapy agents being used (Table 27-1). In clinical practice, patients receiving aggressive chemotherapy have a weekly complete blood count obtained. Dose escalation or reduction can be calculated using nadir counts, which normally occur between 10 and 21 days following treatment. Grading criteria of bone marrow suppression from the Gynecologic Oncology Group is found in Table 27-2.

Neutropenia and Granulocytopenia: Neutropenia (< 3000 WBC/cm^3) and granulocytopenia (< 1500 neutrophils/cm^3) are somewhat arbitrary guidelines commonly used to indicate recovery of internal defenses mediated by WBCs. The absolute neutrophil count (ANC) can be calculated by multiplying the percentage of bands and segmented WBCs by the total WBC (Figure 27-1). Patients receiving either chemotherapy or radiation therapy are at risk to develop life-threatening infections. Although infection would be strongly suspected in patients with fever, neutropenic patients may lack

TABLE 27-1. Selected specific* toxicities leading to laboratory alterations commonly encountered with the use of chemotherapeutic agents in gynecologic oncology

Drug	Toxicity
Amethopterin (Methotrexate)	Myelosuppression Gastrointestinal Hepatic fibrosis and cirrhosis Nephrotoxicity
Carboplatin (Paraplatin)	Hematologic—especially platelets Gastrointestinal Electrolytes
Cisplatin (Platinol)	Gastrointestinal Nephrotoxicity Hypomagnesemia
Cyclophosphamide (Cytoxan)	Gastrointestinal Hematologic—platelet sparing Hemolytic (Coombs'-negative) anemia
Dactinomycin (Cosmegen)	Gastrointestinal Myelosuppression
Doxorubicin (Adriamycin)	Gastrointestinal—hepatically excreted—decrease dose with increased bilirubin
5-Fluorouracil (5-FU, Adrucil, Efudex)	Myelosuppression Gastrointestinal
Hexamethylmelamine (Hexalen, Hexastat)	Nausea and vomiting Myelosuppression
Ifosfamide (IFEX)	Hemorrhagic cystitis—hematuria Myelosuppression Nephrotoxicity
Melphelan (Alkeran)	Myelosuppression
Mitomycin (Mutamycin)	Myelosuppression—watch for late thrombocytopenia (more than 21 days after previous therapy)

Taxol (Paclitaxel)	Myelosuppression
Etoposide VP-16 (Vepesid)	Myelosuppression Gastrointestinal Hepatic damage
Vinblastine (Velban)	Myelosuppression Gastrointestinal Electrolyte imbalance—SIADH
Vincristine (Oncovin)	Electrolyte imbalance—SIADH

*Myelosuppression is common to most agents; specifically affected or spared marrow products are noted.

Gastrointestinal toxicity (nausea, vomiting, diarrhea or stomatitis) can be evidenced by electrolyte abnormalities, anemia of chronic disease or subtle prerenal kidney dysfunction.

Nephrotoxicity often presents with elevation in BUN or creatinine or a decreased creatinine clearance.

Modified from Table 26-4. Copeland LJ, Lewandowski GS. Chemotherapy in gynecologic oncology. In: Rayburn W, Zuspan F, eds. Drug therapy in obstetrics and gynecology, 3rd Edition. New York: CV Mosby Co 1991, pp 431–443.

the ability to generate a febrile response. Laboratory findings of bandemia or a left shift in the differential may be the sole indicator of life-threatening disease. Sepsis needs to be ruled out by culture and careful observation in neutropenic patients with comparatively mild constitutional symptoms such as malaise or subtle mental status changes. Patients with severe neutropenia (ANC < 200) are at great risk of infection from exogenous sources, as well as their own flora. Prophylactic broad-spectrum antibiotics are routinely given in these settings.

Thrombocytopenia: Bleeding and easy bruising are the obvious physical manifestations of thrombocytopenia. A level of 100,000 platelets/mm^3 is generally regarded as an acceptable level at which to resume chemotherapy or to perform elective invasive procedures. Patients demonstrating a level of 20,000 platelets/mm^3 or less are at risk for occult intracranial or intra-abdominal bleeding, and platelet transfusions are commonly used to raise the level above 50,000 platelets/mm^3. Platelet transfusions may also be used in patients with clinically apparent bleeding (from the aerodigestive or genitourinary tracts) whose levels are > 50,000 platelets/mm^3.

Anemia: Commonly encountered in patients with gynecologic malignancies, anemia may be the result of many factors, including chemotherapy

TABLE 27-2. Modified Gynecologic Oncology Group criteria for bone marrow suppression

Toxicity	0	1	2	3	4
WBC	>4.0	3.0–3.9	2.0–2.9	1.0–1.9	<1.0
Platelets	WNL	75K–NL	50K–75K	25K–50K	<25K
Hemoglobin	WNL	10.0–NL	8.0–10.0	6.5–7.9	<6.5
Granulocytes Bands Lymphocytes	>2.0	1.5–1.9	1.0–1.4	0.5–0.9	<0.5
Infection	None	Mild	Moderate	Severe	Life threat

WNL, within normal limits

$$\text{WBC} = 1000 \text{ cells/cm}^3 \quad \text{Differential:} \quad \begin{array}{l} 5 \text{ Bands} \\ 10 \text{ Segs} \\ 50 \text{ Lymphocytes} \\ 35 \text{ Monocytes} \end{array}$$

$$\frac{\text{\# Bands} + \text{\# Segs}}{100 \text{ WBCs}} \times \text{WBC} = \text{ANC} = 1000 \times \frac{5 + 10}{100} = 150$$

FIGURE 27-1. Absolute neutrophil count (ANC)

(bone marrow suppression), radiation effects on bowel resorption, surgical interruption of the bowel (particularly the terminal ileum), occult loss from the gastrointestinal and genitourinary tracts, and phlebotomy. Although the evaluation of peripheral smears, vitamin B_{12}, and folate levels might indicate correctable causes of anemia, the majority of individuals will have a clinical picture consistent with anemia of chronic disease including low serum iron and low total iron-binding capacity (TIBC).

Renal Complications and Electrolyte Disturbances

The close anatomic relationship between the urinary and female reproductive systems explains, in part, the profound effects that gynecologic cancer can have on renal function. Obstructive uropathy can be caused by either direct tumor spread or fibrosis. Immune suppression may contribute to an increased frequency of both lower and upper urinary tract infections.

Dehydration from inadequate fluid intake is often compounded by intravascular volume depletion from vomiting or diarrhea. The depletion in total body protein, which defines the cachetic state commonly encountered in advanced malignancy, lessens the reliability of blood urea nitrogen (BUN) measurements. Serum creatinine and creatinine clearance are more useful in determining dose adjustments and can serve as more reproducible measures of renal function. A BUN creatinine ratio of $> 20:1$ would still be considered an indication of prerenal azotemia; however, a time-trend analysis of these laboratory results in conjunction with a thorough knowledge of each patient's clinical status is probably of greater importance than any single laboratory value. An exception to this would be a rapidly rising serum creatinine indicative of acute renal obstruction. In this case, prompt evaluation and intervention should be initiated to preserve renal function.

Hypomagnesemia is frequently found in patients who have received chemotherapy with cisplatin or carboplatin. Decreased gastrointestinal motility may be an early clinical indicator of this abnormality. Seizures, coma, and other central nervous system manifestations can occur with profound magnesium deficits.

Hepatic Complications

Although the liver parenchyma is a relatively uncommon early site of metastasis for gynecologic tumors, both cancer metastasis and the effects of antineoplastic therapy can result in significant compromise. Liver-associated enzymes are normally not elevated until after metastases have become apparent either through physical examination or imaging studies. Lactate dehydrogenase (LDH) or alkaline phosphatase elevations are often early indicators of metastatic disease. Patients undergoing chemotherapy may eventually demonstrate the changes in glucose and amino acid metabolism found in patients with nonmalignant hepatic disease. Of primary concern are the mental status changes encountered in accumulation of serum ammonia as well as an alteration in coagulation studies including the prothrombin time. Vitamin K-dependent coagulation factors include factors II, VII, IX, and X. Symptomatic bleeding as a result of deficient production of these factors can be temporarily corrected using transfusions of fresh frozen plasma.

Laboratory Assessment of Nutritional Status in Oncology Patients

Nutritional compromise may be secondary to the surgical resection of various lengths of bowel, therapy-related nausea and vomiting, mucosal toxicity, diarrhea, and intestinal malabsorption. A serum albumin level < 3.0 g/dL or total protein level < 5.5 g/dL indicates major malnutrition. A transferrin level of < 170 mg/dL is another index of visceral protein loss. Finally, the patient's immunocompetence can be demonstrated by the determination of a total lymphocyte count (value < 1200 indicates compromise) or by skin testing with specific allergens.

Laboratory Assessment of Patients on Parenteral Nutrition

The clinical impact of the nutritional derangements noted above can be significant. As a result, parenteral hyperalimentation (total parenteral nutrition, TPN) often plays a vital supportive role in the management of patients undergoing therapy. The laboratory tests used to monitor TPN are listed in Table 27-3.

TABLE 27-3. Laboratory tests useful in monitoring patients receiving total parenteral nutrition

Test	*Interval*
CBC with differential, Na, K, Cl, CO_2, BUN, creatinine, glucose, calcium, magnesium, phosphorus, iron, TIBC, serum protein electrophoresis (SPE), cholesterol, triglycerides, PT/PTT, platelets, serum osmolarity, liver-associated enzymes, alkaline phosphatase, bilirubin	Prior to initiation of nutritional support
Na, K, Cl, CO_2, BUN, glucose, creatinine	Daily × 1 w then every M-W-F
CBC (add differential every Monday)	Every M-W-F
Cholesterol, triglycerides, PT/PTT, platelets, magnesium, phosphorus, TIBC, SPE, liver-associated enzymes, osmolarity, alkaline phosphatase, bilirubin	Weekly (Monday)
24-h urine for urea (UUN) and creatinine	With TPN start then weekly
Dipstick urine for glucose/ketones	Every 6 h

PT/PTT, prothrombin time/partial thromboplastin time

Paraneoplastic Syndromes

The paraneoplastic syndromes can be loosely described as clinical or laboratory manifestations of cancer not directly explainable as a result of the disease itself. These conditions are only rarely encountered in gynecologic malignancy. A partial listing of these syndromes with their laboratory abnormalities follows:

1. Syndrome of inappropriate antidiuretic hormone (SIADH) secretion—small cell neuroendocrine tumors and metastatic squamous cancers
   - Hyponatremia (serum sodium < 120 mEq/mL)
   - Urinary sodium (> 20–40 mEq/L)
   - Hypo-osmolarity
2. Hypercalcemia of malignancy—bone metastases, ectopic parathyroid hormone-like substance
   - Hypercalcemia (total calcium > 10.1 mg/dL)
3. Ectopic hormone production

Suggested Reading

Andreoli TE. Disorders of fluid volume, electrolyte and acid base balance. In: Wyngaarden JB, Smith LH Jr, eds. Cecil textbook of medicine, 18th ed. Philadelphia: WB Saunders, 1988:528–558.

Delgado G. Complications related to the nonradiated gastrointestinal tract. In: Delgado G, Smith JP, eds. Management of complications in gynecologic oncology. New York: John Wiley and Sons, 1982:45–98.

Jenson GJ, Bistrian BR. Total parenteral nutrition: which formulation, for which patients? J Crit Illness 1989;4:78–93.

Kaminski MV Jr, ed. Hyperalimentation: a guide for clinicians. New York: Marcel Dekker, 1985.

Mikuta JJ. The gynecologic patient. In: Dudrick, ed. Manual of preoperative and postoperative care. Philadelphia: WB Saunders, 1983:634–647.

Weksler BB, Moore A, Tepler J. Coagulation disorders. In: Andreoli TE, Carpenter CJC, et al eds. Cecil essentials of medicine, 2d ed. Philadelphia: WB Saunders, 1990:394–402.

28.
Gestational Trophoblastic Disease

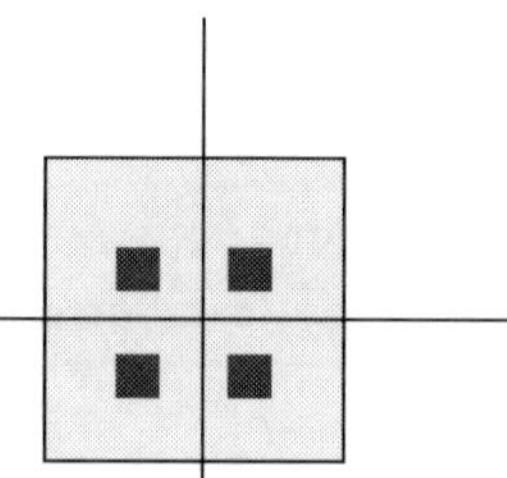

Edward Grendys
James Barter
Willard Barnes

Gestational trophoblastic diseases (GTD) encompass a spectrum of clincopathologic conditions arising from abnormal proliferation of the embryonic trophoblast components. These diseases include complete and partial hydatidiform mole, invasive mole, choriocarcinoma, and placental site trophoblastic tumor (PSTT). Table 28-1 describes these conditions in regard to histologic and cytogenetic differentiation. This chapter focuses on the clinical laboratory testing used in the assessment of these patients.

Human Chorionic Gonadotropin

Hertig described GTD as "God's first cancer and man's first cure" (1). It holds a unique place in oncology history for two reasons. It was the first human malignancy cured with chemotherapy (2) and the first to have an exact, precise serum tumor marker, β-human chorionic gonadotropin (β-hCG), accurately reflecting disease status (3).

Determination of β-hCG levels may help in the initial diagnosis of GTD. High quantitative levels (> 100,000 mIU/mL) obtained from pregnant patients with abnormal bleeding, greater than expected uterine enlargement, absent fetal heart tones, symptoms of hyperemesis, or early pregnancy-induced hypertension may lead to sonographic confirmation of molar pregnancy. Elevated levels in patients with persistent postpartum bleeding may help to diagnose the rare patient developing choriocarcinoma following normal pregnancy.

TABLE 28-1. Gestational trophoblastic disease—histologic and cytogenetic differentiation

Histologic Features	Cytogenetics
Complete Mole	
• Trophoblastic proliferation	Diploid
• Villous edema	46,XX
	46,XY (5–10%)
Partial Mole	
• Less trophoblastic proliferation	Triploid, XXY (60%)
• Mixture of edematous villi with smaller villi 46,XX (rare)	Triploid, XXX (40%)
• Fetal or embryonic tissue and villous vessels may be seen	Triploid, XYY (rare)
Invasive Mole	
• Molar villi outside the endometrial cavity	
Choriocarcinoma	
• Primarily a mixture of cytotrophoblast and syncytiotrophoblast, intermediate trophoblast is also present	
• Usually no villi except for rare cases of development in placenta	
• Tissue invasion, vessel permeation	
• Immunocytochemistry strong for hCG	
Placental Site Trophoblastic Tumor	
• Predominantly intermediate trophoblast showing invasion	
• Immunocytochemistry strong for human placental lactogen	

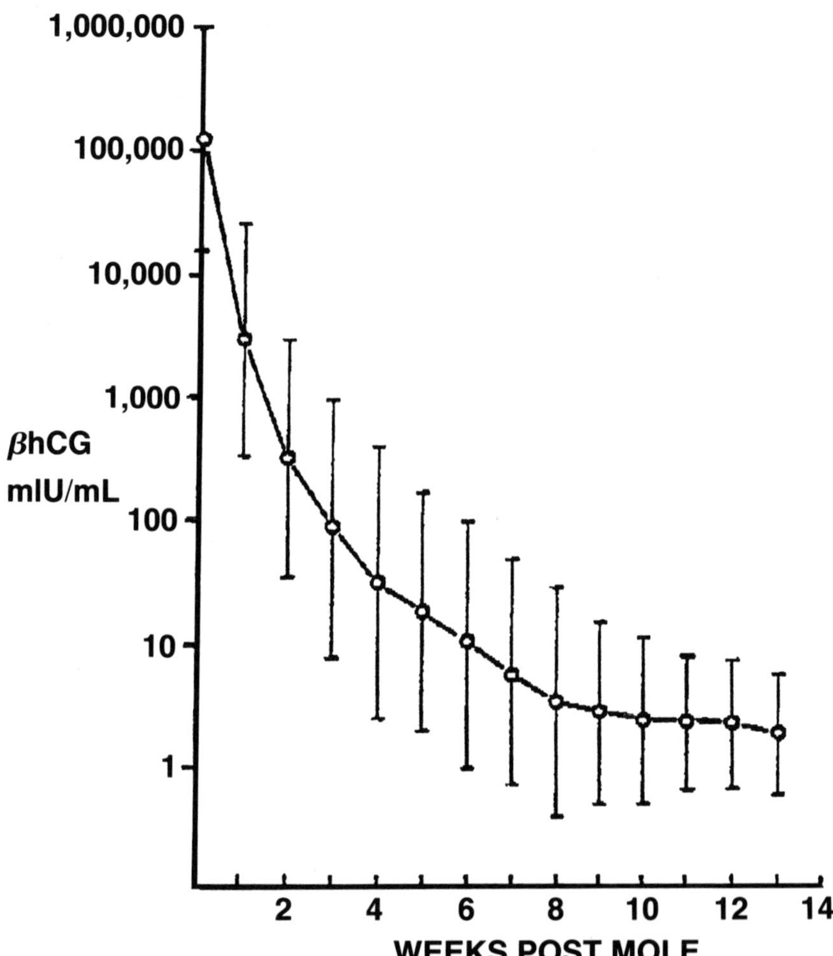

FIGURE 28-1. The mean value and 95% confidence limits describing the normal postmolar β-hCG regression curve. (Reproduced by permission from Schlaerth JB, Morrow CP, Kletsky OA, Nalick RH, D'Ablaing GA. Prognostic characteristics of serum human chorionic gonadotropin titer regression following molar pregnancy. Obstet Gynecol. 1981;58:478–482.)

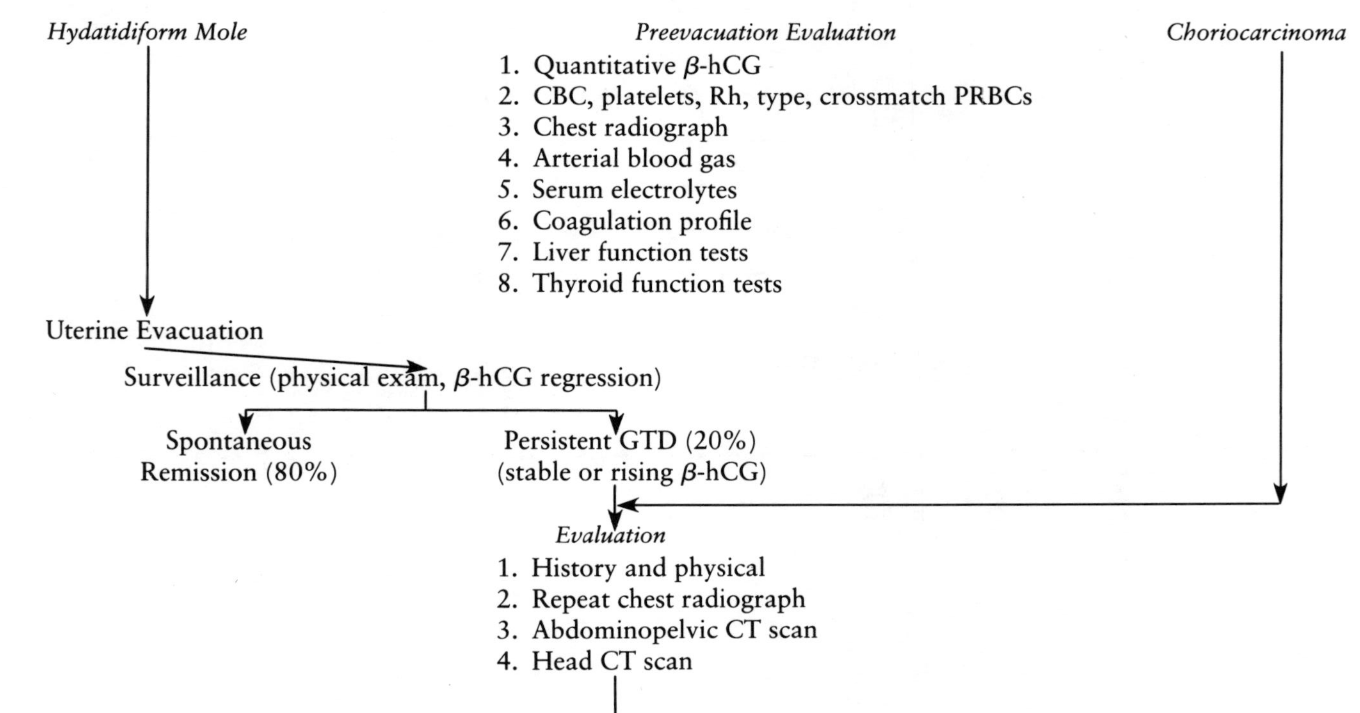

Hydatidiform Mole
Choriocarcinoma
Preevacuation Evaluation
1. Quantitative β-hCG
2. CBC, platelets, Rh, type, crossmatch PRBCs
3. Chest radiograph
4. Arterial blood gas
5. Serum electrolytes
6. Coagulation profile
7. Liver function tests
8. Thyroid function tests
Uterine Evacuation
Surveillance (physical exam, β-hCG regression)
Spontaneous Remission (80%)
Persistent GTD (20%) (stable or rising β-hCG)
Evaluation
1. History and physical
2. Repeat chest radiograph
3. Abdominopelvic CT scan
4. Head CT scan

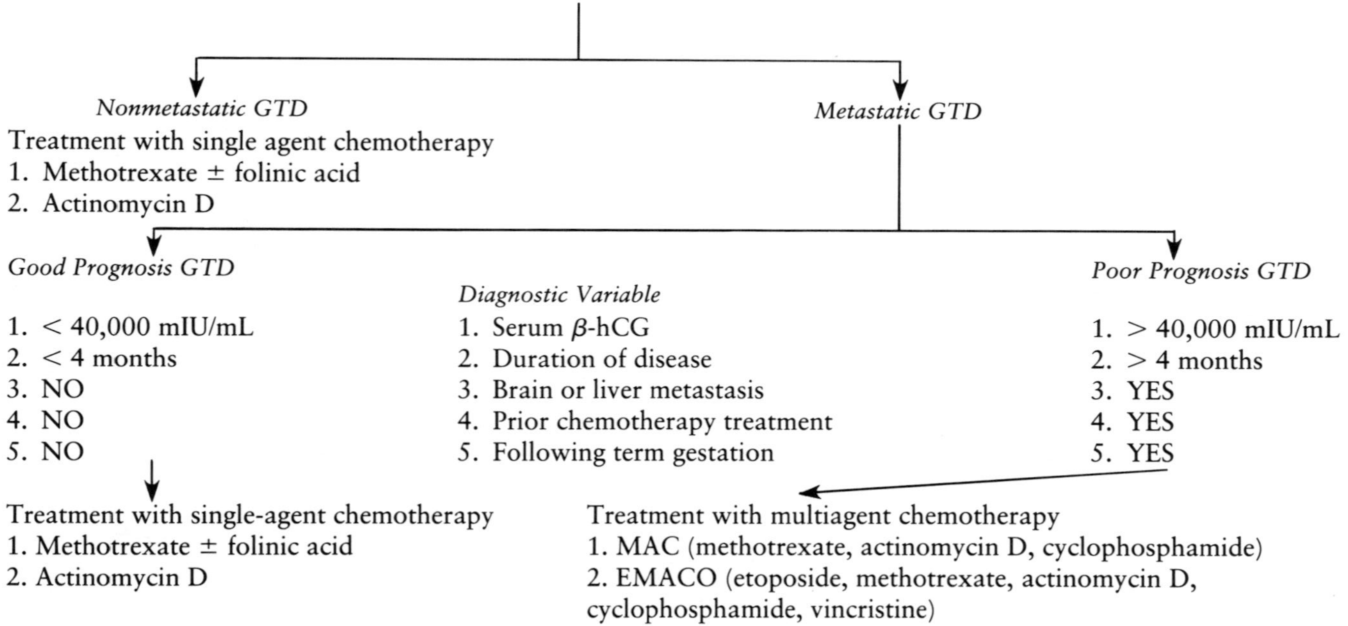

FIGURE 28-2. Management of Gestational Trophoblastic Disease

The level of β-hCG is crucial in management of patients with molar pregnancy following suction curettage. Approximately 20% of evacuated hydatidiform moles may develop into persistent disease as recognized by plateaued or rising hCG levels (4,5). After evacuation, follow-up with weekly serum quantitative β-hCG levels is essential, and these results should be plotted in a semilogarithmic fashion (6; Figure 28-1). In the majority of cases, the postevacuation hCG level will exhibit a progressive decline to normal within 14 weeks of evacuation. Usually when the level is < 100 mIU/mL, a determination of hCG every other week is adequate (7). Prevention of pregnancy (usually with oral contraceptives) is critical for patient management, so that the hCG determinations can be followed.

In addition to identifying patients with persistent disease, quantitative levels are also used to help identify those patients in higher risk groups with metastatic GTD (Figure 28-2). A level > 40,000 mIU/mL is one of the factors that places a patient in the poor prognosis group.

Assessment of β-hCG, however, has not proven helpful in the management of PSTT. This tumor usually produces low hCG levels and thus its use as a clinical marker of disease status is limited. Unlike other forms of GTD, PSTT may be very resistant to chemotherapy. Primary hysterectomy for nonmetastatic disease remains the treatment of choice (8).

Laboratory Evaluation Before Molar Evacuation

Care must be taken perioperatively to minimize potential complications associated with evacuation. Sudden, life-threatening problems may arise and one must not be cavalier in undertaking this procedure. Figure 28-2 lists the laboratory studies suggested *prior* to evacuation to quantitative β-hCG.

Blood Counts, Type, Crossmatch, Rh Status: Hemorrhage may, and often does, occur with evacuation, and 2–4 units of packed red blood cells should be available. Severe preoperative anemia should be corrected before the procedure. In 1980, Goto and colleagues demonstrated Rh-D antigen presence on the molar trophoblast (9). Thus, prophylactic anti-D antibody (Rho-Gam™) should be administered to Rh-negative patients after evacuation to avoid Rh sensitization.

Respiratory Arterial Blood Gas: Approximately 2% of evacuated patients experience acute respiratory distress syndrome, which is probably multifactorial in origin. Pulmonary trophoblastic embolization (10) may occur, although one study revealed only a scant amount of trophoblastic tissue in the pulmonary arterial blood of patients undergoing molar evacuation (11). These investigators concluded that pulmonary complications may result from combined effects of preeclampsia, hyperthyroidism, iatrogenic fluid overload, or anesthetic agents, and therefore, may be preventable. Patients with excessive uterine enlargement ($> 14–16$ weeks estimated gestational age), and markedly elevated hCG levels ($> 100,000$ mIU/mL) are especially at risk for this complication. The patient may experience shortness of breath, tachypnea, and tachycardia, and a chest radiograph will reveal diffuse bilateral infiltrates consistent with respiratory distress syndrome.

Electrolytes: As with any surgical procedure, electrolytes should be evaluated before anesthetic agent use. Electrolyte disturbances are especially common in hyperemetic patients. Perioperative fluid shifts and the antidiuretic hormone effect of oxytocic agents administered during the evacuation mandate careful electrolyte monitoring.

Coagulation Profile: Coagulation cascade abnormalities must be recognized in molar gestation (12). Thromboplastin-like substance deportation with uterine evacuation, especially if $> 14–16$ week size, can lead to rapid disseminated intravascular coagulation, similar to that seen with amniotic fluid embolism. If the platelet count is normal, full evaluation of the coagulation system is usually not necessary.

Liver Function: The liver, a favored site of GTD metastatic spread, also metabolizes many of the commonly used anesthetic agents. Hence, baseline liver functions, alanine transferase, aspartate transferase, alkaline phosphatase, direct and indirect bilirubin, and lactate dehydrogenase are advised.

Endocrine-Thyroid Function Tests: Potentially life-threatening hyperthyroidism (thyrotoxicosis) has been observed in 7% of GTD patients (13). Clinically obvious signs of hyperthyroidism need to be remembered, and if present, confirmed with laboratory studies (thyroid-stimulating hormone, T_3 resin uptake, free T_4) and controlled prior to evacuation. Homology between hCG and the thyroid-stimulating hormone α subunit is the putative cause of thyroid stimulation, although this has not been conclusively proven.

References

1. Hertig AT. Human trophoblast. Springfield, Il: Charles C. Thomas, 1968.
2. Li M, Hertz R, Spencer DB. Effect of methotrexate therapy on choriocarcinoma and chorioadenoma. Proc Soc Exp Biol Med 1956;93:361–366.

3. Vaitukaitis JL, Ross GT, Reichert LE. Immunologic and biologic behavior of hCG and bovine LH subunit hybrids. Endocrinology 1973;92:411–416.

4. Lurain JR, Brewer JI, Torok EE, et al. Natural history of hydatidiform mole after primary evacuation. Am J Obstet Gynecol 1983;145:591–595.

5. Morrow CP. Postmolar trophoblastic disease: diagnosis, management and prognosis. Clin Obstet Gynecol 1984;27:211–220.

6. Morrow CP, Kletzky OA, DiSaia PJ, et al. Clinical and laboratory correlates of molar pregnancy and trophoblastic disease. Am J Obstet Gynecol 1977; 128:424–429.

7. Morrow CP, Townsend D. Tumors of the placental trophoblast. In: Synopsis of gynecologic oncology. New York: Churchill Livingstone, 1987:367.

8. Soper J, Hammond CB, Lewis JL. Gestational trophoblastic disease. In: Hoskins W, Perez C, Young R, eds. Principles and practice of gynecologic oncology. Philadelphia: JB Lippincott, 1992:795–825.

9. Goto S, Nishi H, Tomoda Y. Blood group Rh-D factor in human trophoblast determined by immunofluorescent method. Am J Obstet Gynecol 1980; 137:707–712.

10. Kohorn EI, McGinn RC, Gee JBL, Goldstein DP, Osathanondh R. Pulmonary embolization of trophoblastic tissue in molar pregnancy. Obstet Gynecol 1978;51:16s–20s.

11. Hankins GDV, Wendel GD, Snyder RR, et al. Trophoblastic embolization during molar evacuation: central hemodynamic observations. Obstet Gynecol 1987;69:368–372.

12. Egley CE, Simon LR, Haddox T. Hydatidiform mole and disseminated intravascular coagulation. Am J Obstet Gynecol 1975;121:1122–1123.

13. Amir SM, Osathanondh R, Berkowitz RS, et al. Human chorionic gonadotropin and thyroid function in patients with hydatidiform mole. Am J Obstet Gynecol 1984;150:723–728.

Suggested Reading

Soper JT, Clarke-Pearson DL, Hammond CB. Metastatic gestational trophoblastic disease: Prognostic factors in previously untreated patients. Obstet Gynecol 1988;71:338–43.

Barter JF, Soong SH, Hatch KD, et al. Treatment of non-metastatic gestational trophoblastic disease with oral methotrexate. Am J Obstet Gynecol 1987; 157:1166–68.

Petrilli ES, Twiggs LB, Blessing JA, et al. Single-dose actinomycin D treatment for nonmetastatic gestational trophoblastic disease. A prospective phase II trial of the Gynecologic Oncology Group. Cancer 1987;60:2173–76.

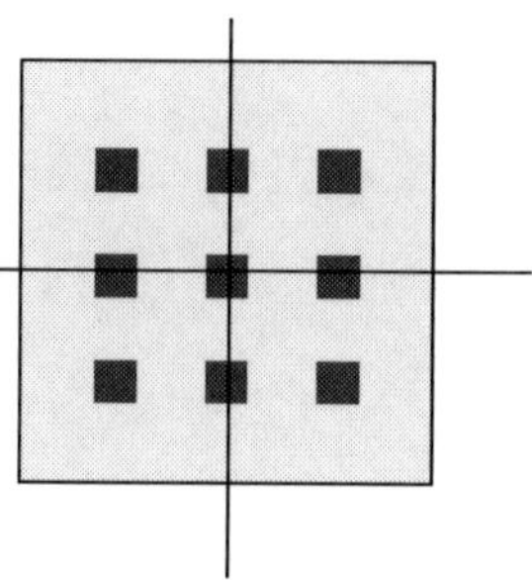

PART SEVEN
Laboratory Tests

ABO DETERMINATION

Specimen Collection: Serum or EDTA

Reference Range: Reported as types A, B, AB, or O

Clinical Correlation: Test interference can occur with recent transfusion, intravenous contrast media, dextran administration, abnormal proteins in the patient's blood, and some cases of bacteremia.

ABO testing is performed:

1. On all pregnant women and all cord blood samples
2. In all situations where a blood transfusion may be required
3. In paternity testing
4. In forensic evaluations (ie, determining secretor status)

ABO incompatibility identified in the nursery occurs more often with group O mothers (production of IgG anti-A and anti-B). Mild hemolytic disease may occur but seldom requires exchange transfusion.

Expected antibodies (anti-A, anti-B) may be absent in some patients with immune deficiencies.

ACETYLCHOLINESTERASE, AMNIOTIC FLUID

Specimen Collection: Amniotic fluid

Reference Range: Negative (abnormal results reported as inconclusive or positive)

Clinical Correlation: Acetylcholinesterase testing is an additional test for neural tube defects (1) that complements evaluation of amniotic fluid α-fetoprotein.

Inconclusive results, though more common prior to 15 weeks' gestation, tend to correlate with anomalies more often after 15 weeks' gestation (2, 3).

Elevated levels may be found in the amniotic fluid of the *unaffected* twin in gestations with diamnionic-monochorionic membranes (4).

Acetylcholinesterase levels are usually normal in trisomies (5).

This test is not dependent on gestational age or affected by fetal bleeding.

A test incorporating the ratio of acetylcholinesterase to pseudocholinesterase has been studied (6). Higher ratios correlate with neural tube defects and are also found in fluid from cystic hygromas. Lower ratios correlate with ventral wall defects, fetal blood, fetal ascites, or a normal outcome.

References

1. Wald NJ, Cuckle HS. Amniotic fluid acetylcholinesterase electrophoresis as a secondary test in the diagnosis of anencephaly and open spina bifida in early pregnancy. Lancet 1981;2:321–327.
2. Drugan A, Syner FN, Belsky R, Koppitch FC 3d, Evans MI. Fluid acetylcholinesterase: implications of an inconclusive result. Am J Obstet Gynecol 1988;159:469–474.
3. Drugan A, Syner FN, Greb A, Evans MI. Amniotic fluid alpha-fetoprotein and acetylcholinesterase in early genetic amniocentesis. Obstet Gynecol 1988; 72:35–38.
4. Stiller RJ, Lockwood CJ, Belanger K, Baumgarten A, Hobbins J, Mahoney MJ. Amniotic fluid alpha-fetoprotein concentrations in twin gestations: dependence on placental membrane anatomy. Am J Obstet Gynecol 1988;158:1088–1092.
5. Buamah PK, Skillen AW, Harrison J, Davison V. Amniotic fluid acetylcholinesterase activity and alpha-fetoprotein in chromosomal anomalies and neural tube defects. Clin Chem 1985;31:614–615.
6. Kelly JC, Petrocik E, Wassman ER. Amniotic fluid acetylcholinesterase ratios in prenatal diagnosis of fetal abnormalities. Am J Obstet Gynecol 1989; 161:703–705.

ACID PHOSPHATASE

Specimen Collection: Vaginal saline lavage or from vaginal fluid-stained clothing fragments (soak in physiologic saline for one hour)

Reference Range: Vaginal acid phosphatase is normally < 10 units/L. Postcoital level is usually > 50 units/L.

Clinical Correlation: This test is applied in evaluation of sexual assault. Small amounts of acid phosphatase may be present in the vaginal secretions of sexually inactive women. Acid phosphatase levels in semen are many times that of vaginal secretion or urine. The decrease in acid phosphatase is variable over time. This test is still useful when the assailant is aspermic or on stained material months old.

Suggested Reading

1. Schumann GB, Badawy S, Peglow A, Henry JB. Prostatic acid phosphatase. Current assessment in vaginal fluid of alleged rape victims. Am J Clin Pathol 1976;66:944–952.
2. Masoods S, Bernhardt HE, Sager N. Quantitative determinations of endogenous acid phosphatase activity in vaginal washings. Obstet Gynecol 1978;51:33–36.

ACTH STIMULATION TEST
Preston Sacks, MD

Specimen Collection
Method 1

1. Serum is obtained for baseline measurement of progesterone (P) and 17 hydroxyprogesterone (17-OHP)
2. 250 μg ACTH 1–24 (Cortrosyn®) is administered intravenously
3. 30 minutes later, serum is obtained for the measurement of P and 17-OHP

The test value is calculated from the formula

$$\frac{(P_{30} \text{ minus } P_0) + (17\text{-}OHP_{30} \text{ minus } 17\text{-}OHP_0)}{30} = ng/dL/min$$

Reference range (for method 1)
Normal is ≤ 6.8 ng/dL/min
Congenital adrenal hyperplasia > 6.8 ng/dL/min

Method 2

1. Serum is obtained for baseline measurement of 17-OHP
2. 250 μg of ACTH 1–24 (Cortrosyn®) is administered intravenously
3. Serum is obtained 60 minutes following ACTH administration for measurement of the stimulated 17-OHP concentration

Reference range (for method 2)
The log of the baseline 17-OHP and log of the stimulated 17-OHP concentrations are plotted on the nomogram created by New (1).

Clinical Correlation: In gynecology this test is usually performed in patients presenting with hirsutism who demonstrate elevated levels of 17-OHP on a single 8 AM screening measurement (2).

References

1. New MI, Lorenzen F, Lerner AJ, et al. Genotyping steroid 21-hydroxylase deficiency: hormonal reference data. J Clin Endocrinol Metab 1983;57:320–326.
2. Azziz R, Zacur HA. 21-hydroxylase deficiency in female hyperandrogenism: screening and diagnosis. J Clin Endocrinol Metab 1989;69:577–584.

Actinomyces

Organism: Anaerobic bacteria (or microaerophilic), gram positive

Specimen Collection: A Pap smear from a patient with an intrauterine device (IUD) may identify actinomyces-like structures.

Pelvic/abdominal abscesses require proper anaerobic culture collection techniques. The rare cases of actinomycotic abscesses are usually related to perforated bowel but can also arise secondary to pelvic inflammation. If a draining sinus has the presence of small yellowish granules (sulfur granules), actinomyces should be suspected. The granules should be sent to the laboratory for identification. When culturing the sinus, it is preferable to collect the specimen as high as possible.

Identification: The major clue to identification is the presence of "sulfur granules," which can be identified grossly and microscopically.

Gram stain—gram-positive branching bacilli identified. Denser staining centrally, with eosinophilic clubbed rays extending from the center.

Silver stains may help to show the branching more distinctly. If attempting to distinguish *Actinomyces* from *Nocardia*, an acid-fast stain can be performed. *Actinomyces* is acid-fast negative, whereas *Nocardia* is partially acid fast. Immunofluorescent staining is also possible with specific antisera.

Culture—difficult to isolate, sometimes requiring up to 2 weeks of anaerobic conditions.

Clinical Correlation: *Actinomyces* species constitute normal flora in the mouth and gastrointestinal tract. In Ob-Gyn, the clinician most often encounters this organism in association with the IUD. Of women with IUDs, this organism is found in approximately 8% (1) and is associated with prolonged use (2).

Eubacterium nodatum (3) is similar in appearance to *Actinomyces israelii* and has been seen in patients with IUDs. Pathogenicity and clinical implications of this discovery await further investigation.

References

1. Hager QWD, Douglas B, Majumudar B. Pelvic colonization with actinomyces in women using intrauterine contraceptive devices. Am J Obstet Gynecol 1979;135:680–684.

2. Mali B, Joshi JV, Wagle U, et al. Actinomyces in cervical smears of women using intrauterine contraceptive devices. Acta Cytol 1986;30:367–371.
3. Hill GB. *Eubacterium nodatum* mimics *Actinomyces* in intrauterine device-associated infections and other settings within the female genital tract. Obstet Gynecol 1992;79:534–538.

ACTIVATED PARTIAL THROMBOPLASTIN TIME (aPTT)

Specimen Collection: Citrate tube

Reference Range: Reagent dependent but usually within the 25–35-second range

Clinical Correlation: The aPTT test evaluates the intrinsic coagulation system. The patient's plasma is first added to an activator (such as kaolin). After the addition of a standardized phospholipid preparation and $CaCl_2$, the time for clot formation is measured.

A prolonged aPTT is found with any of the following:

1. Deficiencies in factors I, II, V, VIII, IX, X, XI, XII (usually < 30% of normal)
2. Inhibitors directed against factors, factor complexes, or phospholipid

If the patient has a normal prothrombin time but prolonged aPTT there is a deficiency in VIII, IX, XI, XII, or an inhibitor present. Inhibitors may be directed against a single factor or against the phospholipid used in the assay (lupus type). See also Lupus Anticoagulant in this section.

If the patient also has a prolonged prothrombin time, the abnormality is in the part of the pathway common to the intrinsic and extrinsic system, namely, I, II, V, and X.

The aPTT is used to monitor heparin therapy. Attempts are made to keep the patient in the 50–70-second range.

The aPTT and prothrombin time should be used for screening of coagulation problems when the patient history suggests prolonged bleeding, easy bruisability, and history of thromboembolic disease.

ALANINE AMINOTRANSFERASE (ALT)

Specimen Collection: Serum

Reference Range: 10–60 units/L

Clinical Correlation: ALT, also termed serum glutamate-pyruvate transaminase (SGPT), is an enzyme found in high amounts in the liver and kidney. Lesser amounts are seen in skeletal muscle and heart. Aminotransferases catalyze amino group transfers between amino acids and α-keto acids. One of the more common uses of this test in Ob-Gyn is to evaluate patients for HELLP (hemolysis, elevated liver enzymes, low platelets) syndrome and as a general assessment of liver injury. The largest elevations will occur in hepatitis. Moderate elevations may be seen in acute fatty liver of pregnancy and mild elevations in cholecystitis and intra-hepatic cholestasis of pregnancy. *Minor* elevations can occur from a large number of diseases and exceedingly long list of medications.

Blood donor testing has incorporated use of ALT to help screen for evidence of hepatitis. The availability now for hepatitis C testing has augmented efforts to prevent posttransfusion hepatitis.

ALBUMIN, SERUM

Specimen Collection: Serum (avoid venostasis when obtaining the specimen)

Reference Range: 3.6–5.2 g/dL (36–52 g/L)
Modest decline occurs with age.

Clinical Correlation: Albumin is the most abundant protein in the plasma and is responsible in large part for the oncotic pressure. It is involved with transport of bilirubin, calcium, cortisol, thyroid hormone, and sex steroids.
Decreased albumin can result from:

1. Decreased synthesis secondary to malnutrition or malabsorption
2. Decreased synthesis secondary to liver disease
3. Increased loss:
    a. Renal (ie, nephrotic syndrome)

b. Skin (ie, burns)

c. Gastrointestinal (ie, protein-losing enteropathy)

4. Catabolic factors (ie, neoplastic, inflammatory)

Serum albumin has been used in the laboratory evaluation of nutritional status in conjunction with total iron-binding capacity, total lymphocyte content, and transferrin. Albumin levels < 3.0 g/dL can be seen in severe malnutrition and may play a role in decisions regarding parenteral nutrition.

Lower albumin levels are noted in pregnancy. This is thought to be related to multiple mechanisms including expanded plasma volume and increased metabolic turnover. Albumin levels of 3.0 g/dL are not uncommonly found at term.

ALCOHOL, BLOOD

Specimen Collection: Clotted or anticoagulated blood can be used; *avoid alcohol swab* prior to blood collection.

Reference Range: Negative. (Intoxication at 50–100 mg/dL, fatalities at > 400 mg/dL)

Clinical Correlation: Ethanol is of concern in pregnancy in terms of fetal alcohol syndrome, its direct toxicity, and injuries incurred secondary to its systemic effects.

ALKALINE PHOSPHATASE (AND ISOENZYMES)

Specimen Collection: Serum

Reference Range: 42–98 units/L age 20–60 years
53–141 units/L age > 60 years

Isoenzymes: Alkaline phosphatase isoenzymes include the following:

1. *Liver*—Two fractions have been described. One fraction contributes to the significant elevation of alkaline phosphatase in intrahepatic and extrahepatic obstructive disease. Another fraction, which is noted to have slow migration in starch and polyacrylamide gel, is seen more often in liver parenchymal disease.

2. *Bone*—The fraction from bone can be elevated in many conditions associated with increased osteoblastic activity.

3. *Intestinal*—This fraction can be elevated after a meal, especially with individuals with type O and B blood types.
4. *Placental*—This fraction's contribution causes nearly a doubling of alkaline phosphatase in pregnancy. This isoenzyme is heat stable.
5. *Tumor associated*—These isoenzymes include Regan, Nagao, Kasahara, and hepatoma.

Clinical Correlation: During pregnancy, levels rise in the first and second trimester and peak in the third trimester to about twice the normal non-pregnant level, due to contribution by placental alkaline phosphatase, which makes up approximately 40% to 65% of the total enzyme amount.

The use of alkaline phosphatase is limited in Ob-Gyn. Marked elevations above the normally seen increase in pregnancy may be seen in acute fatty liver of pregnancy, intrahepatic cholestasis, and in biliary tract disease.

α-FETOPROTEIN, AMNIOTIC FLUID (AF-AFP)

Specimen Collection: Amniotic fluid
Specimen contamination with fetal blood alters results.

Reference Range: As with maternal serum, the amniotic fluid level of AFP is converted to multiples of the median (MOM) and significant levels are in the 2.0–2.5 MOM range (or above).

In normal pregnancy the amniotic fluid AFP increases until 14 weeks and then decreases by approximately 10% per week.

It is very important to recognize that each laboratory sets its own reference range.

Clinical Correlation: Principally used in the diagnosis of neural tube defects. Amniotic fluid acetylcholinesterase determinations are performed additionally when AF-AFP levels are elevated.

A slide test for AFP has been used to help diagnose rupture of the membranes (1).

Reference

1. Rochelson BL, Rodke G, White R, Bracero L, Baker DA. A rapid colorimetric AFP monoclonal antibody test for the diagnosis of preterm rupture of the membranes. Obstet Gynecol 1987;69:163–166.

α-FETOPROTEIN (AFP), SERUM

Specimen Collection: Serum

Reference Range: Adult nonpregnant level is < 15 ng/mL.

Normal pregnancy level rises 15% per week until 30 weeks, followed by a 4-week plateau and then steady decline.

Clinical Correlation: Maternal serum α-fetoprotein (MSAFP) has diagnostic utility in the following:

1. Detection of neural tube defects (NTD) and other congenital problems (cystic hygroma, ventral wall defects, nephrosis, etc)
2. Prenatal risk assessment for some trisomies

Division of the patient's MSAFP serum concentration by the median value from a normal pregnancy and adjusted for weight, race, and diabetes produces a value called multiple of the median or MOM. Risk for NTD and other congenital problems is higher when the patient's MOM value is in the 2.0–2.5 range (or above). 0.5% of *normal* pregnancies have AFP above 2.5 multiples of the median (MOM).

Significantly decreased AFP values (< 0.4 MOM) are associated with an increase risk for Down syndrome. AFP is used in conjunction with human chorionic gonadotropin and unconjugated estriol in the "triple screen," which provides a better risk estimate than using AFP alone.

MSAFP elevations are also associated with premature delivery, low birth weight, preeclampsia, and placental abruption.

MSAFP has been used to evaluate evidence of fetomaternal transfusion in patients undergoing chorionic villus sampling (1).

Serum AFP is elevated in germ cell tumors with yolk sac differentiation (yolk sac tumor, embryonal) and is useful as a tumor marker to monitor therapy.

Reference

1. Shulman LP, Meyers CM, Simpson JL, Andersen RN, Tolley EA, Elias S. Fetomaternal transfusion depends on amount of chorionic villi aspirated but not on method of chorionic villus sampling. Am J Obstet Gynecol 1990;162: 1185–1188.

AMINOGLYCOSIDE ASSAYS

Amikacin

Specimen Collection: Serum, draw ½ hour prior to dose for trough, ½–1 hour after dose for peak level

Reference Range:

Therapeutic	peak	15–30 µg/mL
Therapeutic	trough	5–10 µg/mL
Toxic	peak	>35 µg/mL
Toxic	trough	>10 µg/mL

Gentamicin

Specimen Collection: Serum, draw blood for peak level 30 minutes after the end of intravenous infusion, draw blood for trough level just prior to next infusion.

Reference Range:

Therapeutic	peak	6–10 µg/mL
Therapeutic	trough	0.5–1.5 µg/mL
Toxic	peak	>12–15 µg/mL
Toxic	trough	>2 µg/mL

Tobramycin

Specimen Collection: Serum, draw peak sample 30 minutes after dosing, draw trough level immediately before next dose.

Reference Range

Therapeutic	peak	5–10 µg/mL
Therapeutic	trough	1–1.5 µg/mL
Toxic	peak	12 µg/mL

Clinical Correlation: Aminoglycoside levels are usually drawn about 24–36 hours into therapy. Laboratory studies used in evaluation of nephrotoxicity include serum creatinine, creatinine clearance, and urinary microglobulin. If the patient is on prolonged therapy, drug levels should be monitored every 3–4 days. Body weight and renal status must be carefully considered before initial dosing.

Suggested Reading

Blanco JD, Gibbs RS, Duff P, et al. Serum tobramycin levels in puerperal women. Am J Obstet Gynecol 1983;147:466–468.

Duff P, Jorgensen JH, Alexander G, et al. Serum gentamicin levels in patients with post-cesarean endomyometritis. Obstet Gynecol 1983;61:723–727.

Zaske DE, Cipolle RJ, Strate RG, et al. Rapid gentamicin elimination in obstetric patients. Obstet Gynecol 1980;56:559–563.

AMNIOTIC FLUID-ΔOD_{450}

Specimen Collection: Amniotic fluid from amniocentesis, protect from light exposure, meconium and blood can alter results.

Reference Range and Clinical Correlation: See Chapter 8 on erythroblastosis fetalis.

AMNIOTIC FLUID GRAM STAIN/CULTURE

Specimen Collection: Amniotic fluid from pressure catheter, amniocentesis, or obtained at time of cesarean section

Clinical Correlation: A polymicrobial pattern of organisms (anaerobic/aerobic) can be found if amniotic fluid is cultured at the time of cesarean section (ruptured membranes > 6 hours; 1)

See also Chapter 5 on bacterial infections.

Reference

1. Gilstrap LC III, Cunningham FG. The bacterial pathogenesis of infection following cesarean section. Obstet Gynecol 1979;53:545.

AMNIOTIC FLUID-OPTICAL DENSITY-FETAL MATURITY

Specimen Collection: Amniotic fluid
Blood, meconium, and bilirubin can interfere with test results.

Reference Range: Optical density > 0.15 has been correlated with mature lecithin/sphingo-myelin ratio.

Clinical Correlation: The test is based on turbidity changes from surfactant lamellae.
Hydramnios may have decreased turbidity secondary to dilutional effect.

Suggested Reading

Cetrulo CL, Sbarra AJ, Selvaraj RJ, et al. Positive correlation between mature amniotic fluid optical density readings and the absence of neonatal hyaline membrane disease. J Reprod Med 1985;30:929–932.

Slothouber JH, Flu PK, Wallenburg HC. Relationship between amniotic fluid optical density and L/S ratio. J Perinat Med 1987;15:239–243.

Tsai MY, Josephson MW, Knox GE. Absorbance of amniotic fluid at 650 nm as a fetal lung maturity test: a comparison with the lecithin/sphingomyelin ratio and tests for desaturated phosphatidylcholine and phosphatidylglycerol. Am J Obstet Gynecol 1983;146:963–966.

AMYLASE, SERUM AND URINE

Specimen collection: Serum
Urine (timed collections of 1, 2 or 24 hours, no preservative)

Reference Range: Serum—(11–128 units/L)
Urine—17 units/L per hour

Clinical Correlation: Serum amylase determination represents the measurement of different isoenzymes derived from the pancreas, salivary glands, and fallopian tube with minor contribution from other organs. Primary use of the test by Ob-Gyn physicians is the diagnosis of pancreatitis in women presenting with abdominal pain. With pancreatitis, serum amylase levels are usually at least three times normal. Serum lipase is usually ordered in conjunction with amylase.

The urine amylase may sometimes remain elevated in pancreatitis when the serum amylase is returning to normal levels (time lag 6–10 hours).

Although it may rarely be elevated in ectopic pregnancies, serum amylase is not considered a diagnostic test for ectopic pregnancy.

Only rare cases of ovarian cancer have manifested elevated serum amylase levels.

Pancreatitis should be suspected in the postoperative patient with significantly elevated amylase determinations. Manipulation of the pelvic organs and especially the fallopian tube at the time of surgery does not cause a significant amylase elevation (1).

Reference

1. Frohlich EP, Herz C, van der Merwe FJ, Schein M, Smyth AE. Serum amylase levels after obstetric and gynecologic operations. Surg Gynecol Obstet 1990; 170:292–294.

ANAEROBIC CULTURE TECHNIQUE

Specimen Collection: Specimens include tissue, abscess material, body fluid, blood. Use specimen containers provided by the laboratory. If using a capped syringe, expel the air. Send specimen to the laboratory immediately. Do not submit superficial vaginal or cervical specimens for anaerobic evaluation.

Multiple lumen catheters have been used to obtain anaerobic specimens from the endometrial cavity (1).

Reference

1. Knuppel RS, Scerbo JC, Mitchell GW, et al. Quantitative transcervical uterine cultures with a new device. Obstet Gynecol 1981;57:243–248.

ANTIBODY TITER

Specimen Collection: Serum

Reference Range: Negative

Clinical Correlation: Dilutional titers can be performed to determine the relative strength of an antibody in the serum. This is determined for Rh and irregular antibodies detected on antibody screening. See Chapter 8 on erythroblastosis fetalis.

ANTICARDIOLIPIN ANTIBODY (ACA)

Specimen Collection: Serum

Reference Range: Reported in units as:

negative
low positive
medium positive
high positive

Clinical Correlation: ACAs along with lupus anticoagulant are antiphospholipid antibodies. High levels of ACA have been associated with fetal loss and thrombotic complications. This antibody is more commonly seen in patients with systemic lupus erythematosus, especially in those who also demonstrate thrombocytopenia.

Lockwood and colleagues found ACA to be present in 2.2% in a general obstetric population.

Suggested Reading

Lockshin MD, Druzin ML, Goei S, et al. Antibody to cardiolipin as a predictor of fetal distress or death in pregnant patients with systemic lupus erythematosus. N Engl J Med 1985;313:152–156.

Lockwood CJ, Romero R, Feinberg RF, Clyne LP, Coster B, Hobbins JC. The prevalence and biologic significance of lupus anticoagulant and anticardiolipin antibodies in a general obstetric population. Am J Obstet Gynecol 1989;161: 369–373.

ANTICONVULSANTS

Specimen Collection: Serum, plasma (blood drawn just prior to dosing)

Reference Range:

Phenytoin	Therapeutic	10–20 µg/mL
Phenytoin free level	"	1–2 µg/mL
Phenytoin	Toxic (nystagmus)	> 20 µg/mL
Phenytoin	Toxic (decreased mental capacity)	> 40 µg/mL
Carbamazepine	Therapeutic	4–12 µg/mL*
Carbamazepine	Toxic (blurred vision nystagmus, diplopia drowsiness)	>15 µg/mL
Phenobarbital	Therapeutic	15–40 µg/mL
Phenobarbital	Toxic (ataxia nystagmus)	35–70 µg/mL
Phenobarbital	Toxic (coma)	> 65–70 µg/mL
Primadone	Therapeutic	5–12 µg/mL†
Primadone	Toxic (nystagmus sedation, ataxia)	> 15 µg/mL
Ethosuximide	Therapeutic	40–100 µg/mL
Ethosuximide	Toxic (nausea vomiting, headache dizziness)	> 150 µg/mL

SI conversion factors to convert to µmol/L

Phenytoin × 4
Carbamazepine × 4.2
Phenobarbital × 4.3
Primadone × 4.6
Ethosuximide × 7

* Therapeutic range lower, if patient is on other anticonvulsants
† Phenobarbital is a metabolite and should also be measured

ANTIGLOBULIN TEST, DIRECT

Specimen Collection: EDTA, serum
Important to submit clinical, transfusion, and medication history to the laboratory

Reference Range: Negative

Clinical Correlation: This test is also called the direct Coombs' test. Its purpose is to detect antibody or complement on the red cell surface. The antihuman globulin used to detect coated red cells may be either poly-specific or monospecific (ie, directed just to IgG or directed just a certain complement component). If the red cells are coated, the addition of the antihuman globulin will cause agglutination. Before the red cells are tested, they are washed to remove unbound protein. Direct antiglobulin tests are performed on the following:

1. Red cells of the infant to confirm transfer of maternal antibody
2. Red cells from the patient who has a transfusion reaction
3. Red cells from a patient suspected to have autoimmune hemolytic anemia

A positive direct antiglobulin test can result secondary to medications. Medications used in Ob-Gyn include penicillins, cephalosporins, sulfona-mides, tetracyclines, mefenamic acid, and α-methyldopa.

ANTIGLOBULIN TEST, INDIRECT

Specimen Collection: Serum

Reference Range: Negative

Clinical Correlation: This test helps to determine if any other antibodies (aside from anti-A or anti-B) are present in the serum. Synonyms for this test are antibody screen and indirect Coombs' test. It is important to know if antibodies are present in the following specimens:

1. Serum of a patient who may receive a blood product transfusion
2. Donor serum
3. The serum of a patient who has a transfusion reaction
4. The serum of a pregnant patient

Knowledge of antibodies in the serum guides the blood bank in being able to provide appropriate crossmatched antigen-negative compatible units in case of bleeding complications. Serum antibody evaluation at the initial prenatal examination helps to identify maternal antibodies that may cause hemolytic disease of the newborn.

Type and (antibody) screen procedures usually takes approximately 45 minutes. If an unusual antibody is found, identification may take several days. *Type and screen* testing has replaced *type and crossmatch* for most Ob-Gyn procedures. Type and crossmatch is still important prior to radical gynecologic oncology procedures, suction curettage of molar pregnancies, and obstetric situations with a high risk for major hemorrhage.

ANTIMICROBIAL SUSCEPTIBILITY TESTING

Clinical Correlation: Antimicrobial susceptibility testing is indicated for clinically significant organisms with unpredictable response to antimicrobials. Susceptibility testing should focus on the organism most likely responsible for the clinical infection as opposed to probable contaminants or normal flora.

Dilution and disk diffusion tests, which are the most common methods, evaluate for minimum inhibitory concentration (MIC) of the antimicrobial that will inhibit the organism's growth. Results are listed as sensitive, moderately sensitive, and resistant.

The indications for antimycobacterial and antifungal susceptibility testing are limited.

Another susceptibility test that measures the lethality of the antimicrobial provides results as a minimum bactericidal concentration (MBC). This testing is generally reserved for serious infections in sites where the body's defense capabilities may be more limited (ie, meningitis, osteomyelitis).

Measurement of β-lactamase production is an important laboratory determination that guides antimicrobial therapy. This is important for such organisms such as *Staphylococcus aureus, Neisseria gonorrhoeae, Bacteroides fragilis,* and *Bacteroides disiens.*

Suggested Reading

Washington JA. *In vitro* testing of antimicrobial agents. In: Henry JB, ed. Clinical diagnosis and management by laboratory methods, 18th ed. Philadelphia: WB Saunders, 1991.

ANTINUCLEAR ANTIBODY (ANA)

Specimen Collection: Serum

Reference Range: Titer < 1:32 is negative.

Clinical Correlation: Initial screening test for collagen vascular disease, lacks specificity.

Anti-DNA is used for diagnosis and monitoring of systemic lupus. Along with anti-Smith antibody, it is more specific for lupus.

ANTI-SS-A (Ro) AND ANTI-SS-B (La)

Specimen Collection: Serum

Reference Range: Negative

Clinical Correlation: Anti-SS-A (Ro) is found in approximately 70% of patients with Sjögren's syndrome and 40% of patients with systemic lupus, is associated with neonatal lupus and congenital heart block in the fetus.

Anti-SS-B (La) is found in approximately 50% of patients with Sjögren's syndrome and 10% of patients with systemic lupus, is associated with neonatal lupus and congenital heart block in the fetus.

Suggested Reading

Scott JS, Maddison PJ, Tayler PV, et al. Connective-tissue-disease, antibodies to ribonucleoprotein and congenital heart block. N Engl J Med 1983;309:209–212.

Steier JA, Akslen LA, Flesland O, Askvik K. Fetal heart block, anti-SSA and anti-SSB antibodies. Association with intra-uterine growth retardation, fetal death and lupus anticoagulant. Acta Obstet Gynecol Scand 1987;66:737–739.

Veille JC, Sunderland C, Bennett RM. Complete heart block in a fetus associated with maternal Sjögren's syndrome. Am J Obstet Gynecol 1985;151:660–661.

Watson WJ, Katz VL. Steroid therapy for hydrops associated with antibody-mediated congenital heart block. Am J Obstet Gynecol 1991;165:553–554.

ANTITHROMBIN III

Specimen Collection: Plasma, (citrate tube) place on ice and immediately transport to the laboratory

Reference Range: 21–30 mg/dL (210–300 mg/L) or may be expressed as a percentage of normal

Clinical Correlation: Antithrombin III establishes a coagulation balance by its inactivation of thrombin. Hereditary antithrombin III deficiency is found in 1:2000 to 1:20,000 individuals. Affected individuals with a deficiency of antithrombin III (autosomal dominant) are predisposed to developing thrombotic complications. Conard and coworkers have described this disease in relation to pregnancy (1).

Low levels of antithrombin III interfere with obtaining an adequate anticoagulant response with heparin.

See also Chapter 2 on hypertension for its use in differentiating chronic hypertension from preeclampsia.

Reference

1. Conard J, Horellou MH, Van Dreden P, Lecompte T, Samama M. Thrombosis and pregnancy in congenital deficiencies in AT III, protein C or protein S: study of 78 women. Thromb Haemost 1990;63:319.

ANTITHYROGLOBULIN ANTIBODY

Specimen Collection: Serum

Reference Range: Normal titer is < 1:10.

Clinical Correlation: This test should be considered in the patient presenting with premature ovarian failure. Patients with other autoimmune disorders and normal elderly women may be positive for antibody.

APT TEST

Specimen Collection: Mix bloody fluid with 5–10 parts tap water, centri-
fuge for 2 minutes, mix 5 parts of the pink supernatant with one part 1%
NaOH, and repeat centrifugation.

Reference Range: A pink color indicates fetal blood; a yellow brown
color is indicative of maternal origin.

Clinical Correlation: This test has been used to help determine if fetal
bleeding has occurred with a bloody tap or vaginal bleeding is secondary
to a vasa previa. Fetal hemoglobin is more resistant to denaturation with
alkali than is the adult hemoglobin from a maternal source. Used in conjunction with careful fetal monitoring, this test takes approximately 5
minutes to perform. The use of Wright staining to look for nucleated red
blood cells has also been suggested as a rapid test to assess bleeding origin.

Reference

Apt L, Downey WS. "Melena" neonatorum: the swallowed blood syndrome. J
    Pediatr 1955;47:6.

ARTERIAL BLOOD GASES

Specimen Collection: Arterial puncture, prior Allen test, avoid air in
specimen, heparinized glass syringe, immerse syringe in ice, immediate
transport to laboratory, pressure to puncture site.

Excess heparin can decrease pCO_2, pH will decrease if specimen not
chilled, exposure to room air will lead to increase in measured pO_2.

Tests and Reference Ranges:

	Nonpregnant	*Pregnant*
pO_2	75–100 mm Hg	104–108 mm Hg
pCO_2	35–45 mm Hg	27–32 mm Hg
pH	7.35–7.45	7.35–7.45
O_2 sat	95–99%	95–99%
HCO_3	22–28 mEq/L	18–25 mEq/L

Clinical Correlation: Clinically used in cases of respiratory distress, altered consciousness, metabolic disorders, and shock.

ASPARTATE AMINOTRANSFERASE (AST)

Specimen Collection: Serum

Reference Range: 10–42 units/L

Clinical Correlation: AST is an enzyme found in many areas of the body including heart, liver, skeletal muscle, kidney, brain, pancreas, and lungs. Aminotransferases catalyze amino group transfers between amino acids and α-keto acids. This test is a relatively nonspecific indicator of conditions resulting in cell injury. One of the more frequent uses in Ob-Gyn is to assess the liver in preeclampsia (HELLP syndrome—hemolysis, elevated liver enzymes, low platelets).

In general alanine aminotransferase (ALT) levels are more specific for liver abnormalities than AST levels. The most marked elevations of the aminotransferases are seen in hepatitis, moderate elevations in acute fatty liver of pregnancy, and mild elevations in cholecystitis and intrahepatic cholestasis of pregnancy.

Similar to ALT, *minor* elevations of AST are seen secondary to a multitude of conditions and medications.

Bacteroides bivius, B disiens, B fragilis

Organisms: Obligate anaerobes

Specimen Collection: Anaerobic collection

Clinical Correlation: These anaerobic organisms have been isolated in cases of intra-amniotic infection, postpartum endometritis, bacteremia, and pelvic inflammatory disease. *B fragilis* is occasionally found in the vaginal flora but to much less of a degree than *B bivius* and *B disiens*.

Suggested Reading

Blanco JD, Gibbs RS, Castaneda YS. Bacteremia in obstetrics: clinical course. Obstet Gynecol 1981;58:62.

Gibbs RS, Forman J, St. Clair PJ, Baseman JB. Detection of serum antibody response to *Bacteroides bivius* by enzyme-linked immunosorbent assay in women with intraamniotic infection. Obstet Gynecol 1987;69:208–213.

Kirby BD, George WL, Sutter VL, Citron DM, Finegold SM. Gram-negative anaerobic bacilli: their role in infection and patterns of susceptibility to antimicrobial agents. I. Little-known *Bacteroides* species. Rev Infect Dis 1980;2:914.

Snydman DR, Tally FP, Knuppel R, et al. *Bacteroides bivius* and *Bacteroides disiens* in obstetrical patients: clinical findings and antimicrobial susceptibilities. J Antimicrob Chemother 1980;6:519–525.

BILE ACIDS

Specimen Collection: Serum, usually postprandial specimen drawn

Reference Range: Total 3–30 mg/L (0.8–8.0 µmol/L)

Clinical Correlation: A slight increase in levels has been seen in normal pregnancy. Total bile acids are significantly elevated in intrahepatic cholestasis of pregnancy. Modest elevations of bilirubin, alkaline phosphatase, and aminotransferases are also noted in this condition.

Suggested Reading

Lunzer M, Barnes P, Byth K, O'Halloran M. Serum bile acid concentrations during pregnancy and their relationship to obstetric cholestasis. Gastroenterology 1986;91:825–829.

BILIRUBIN, SERUM

Specimen Collection: Serum

Reference Range:

Direct (conjugated)	0–0.2 mg/dL (0–3.4 µmol/L)
Indirect (unconjugated)	0.1–1.0 mg/dL (1.7–17 µmol/L)
Total	0.2–1.5 mg/dL (3.4–25.7 µmol/L)

Clinical Correlation: Bilirubin is used diagnostically in hepatic diseases and hemolytic anemia. Increased levels of indirect bilirubin are found in hemolytic disease and with hepatic parenchymal damage. Direct bilirubin is elevated in biliary obstruction (ie, intrahepatic cholestasis of pregnancy).

There is no significant change in bilirubin during normal pregnancy.

BLEEDING TIME

Specimen Collection: Duke method from ear lobe is not commonly performed anymore.

Ivy and Mielke (template) methods are from the forearm.

Do not perform if recent aspirin ingestion or significantly low platelets are noted.

Sphygmomanometer measurement of 40 mm Hg is obtained with blood pressure cuff prior to incision. Filter paper is used to blot.

Reference Range: Normal range for Ivy method is 2–7 minutes. It may extend slightly longer with the template methods. Values > 11 minutes are of concern.

Clinical Correlation: Although abnormal in some other rare diseases, von Willebrand's disease would be the most common application for this test for the Ob-Gyn physician.

BLOOD CULTURE

Specimen Collection: The skin should be carefully prepared with alcohol and povidone-iodine sponges. Draw 10–20 mL blood, change needles, and then add blood to aerobic and anaerobic bottles (1:5–1:10 dilution). Note any recent antibiotic use on laboratory slip.

Clinical Correlation: Septicemia in Ob-Gyn can occur in a number of circumstances related to pregnancy complications, pelvic inflammations, and neoplastic disease. Gram-negative bacilli are the predominant organisms found.

Other laboratory parameters evaluated in the septic patient include:

1. Cultures to determine source of infection
2. CBC (the white cell count may be initially decreased)

3. Platelets, fibrinogen, and fibrin degradation products to assess for disseminated intravascular coagulation
4. Arterial blood gases
5. Electrolytes
6. Creatinine and blood urea nitrogen
7. Lactic acid

BLOOD TRANSFUSION

Specimen Collection and Laboratory Testing: After donor screening and collection, the following laboratory studies are performed: ABO-Rh, antibody screen, hepatitis B surface antigen, hepatitis B core antibody, alanine aminotransferase, hepatitis C, antibodies to HIV-1, HIV-2, HTLV-1, and syphilis testing.

Storage and Processing: Blood is commonly combined with a citrate-phosphate-dextrose-adenine solution and stored at 4°C. The shelf life is 35 days. With storage there is a decrease in 2,3-diphosphoglycerate and an increase in potassium.

Transmission of Infection: The "window period" in which HIV-positive, antibody-negative blood may be donated is estimated to extend to around 14 weeks following infection. The chance for an individual patient to receive HIV-positive blood from a single unit is 1:150,000.

Though rare, bacterial contamination of blood and blood products can occur both in homologous and autologous donations. The source of the contamination can be already present in the donor or can occur during the processing and storage of the product. Gram-negative organisms are more common. Pseudomonas has been found in approximately a fourth of the cases.

Transfusion Reactions: *Hemolytic reactions*—Hemolytic reaction can be immediate or delayed. The most common acute hemolytic transfusion reaction is secondary to ABO-incompatible blood. An anticoagulated and clot specimen are drawn. The appearance of a pink color in the plasma or serum indicates intravascular hemolysis. Other (less immediate) laboratory studies that are indicative of hemolysis include increased indirect bilirubin, decreased haptoglobin, and hemoglobinuria. If hemolysis is confirmed, repeat type and crossmatch is performed on pre- and posttransfusion specimens. Pre- and posttransfusion serum is tested against red cell panels in an effort to identify antibodies. Special techniques may be needed to improve antibody detection. The direct antiglobulin test is performed to identify antibody coating. Blood urea nitrogen, creatinine, and electrolyte levels should be carefully monitored.

Anaphylactic—Laboratory evaluation of a patient with immediate generalized reaction might disclose the rare patient deficient in IgA.

Citrate toxicity—Rapid transfusions can cause decreased levels of ionized calcium secondary to the chelating properties of citrate. Potassium levels can vary in massive transfusions. Potassium in banked blood increases with storage time. The metabolism of citrate, however, can lead to alkalosis and subsequent hypokalemia.

Febrile reactions—Leukoagglutinins are implicated in these reactions. Perform laboratory evaluation to rule out a hemolytic reaction. If fever and shock occur, it is important to look for evidence of contaminated donor blood. Gram stain and culture of pre- and posttransfusion blood should be performed.

Graft-versus-host disease—In Ob-Gyn this situation occurs mainly in intrauterine transfusions. This complication is prevented by irradiating the blood before transfusion.

Clinical Correlation: It is estimated that about 2% of women require blood transfusion in the peripartum time period (1).

Whole blood and modified whole blood (minus cryoprecipitate or platelets) are not used or available in many areas. The use of packed red cells and specific components has supplanted the use of whole blood in most situations. Use of packed red cells lessens the chance of nonhemolytic reactions due to the smaller quantities of white cells and isohemoagglutinins. If whole blood is available, the clinician could consider its use in massive transfusions where the added coagulation factors and proteins may help in management.

For most elective procedures, type and screen is adequate before the procedure. Type and crossmatch testing is used before radical gynecologic operations, curettage of molar pregnancies, and certain obstetric conditions with a high risk for bleeding at the time of delivery. If blood is needed quickly and the patient has already had a type and screen, it takes a few minutes to perform an "immediate spin" crossmatch.

In life-threatening situations, uncrossmatched blood may need to be given to a patient. Group specific or group O Rh-negative blood should be given to the woman in this circumstance.

Directed donation allows a patient to select donors, usually family and friends, to provide blood for exclusive use by the patient. The donated blood is subjected to the same testing. Studies have not indicated any increased safety over and above that of general banked blood (2). Some benefit may be accrued if it helps with patient anxiety.

General principles guiding the use of blood transfusion encourage the clinician to transfuse only when clinical parameters require it. With massive transfusions careful monitoring of CBC, platelets, prothrombin time, and partial thromboplastin time guides blood and component therapy.

The use of hemodilution techniques is one of the few methods that can be provided to Jehovah's Witnesses.

References

1. Klapholz H. Blood transfusion in contemporary obstetric practice. Obstet Gynecol 1990;75:940–943.
2. Starkey JM, et al. Markers for transfusion-transmitted disease in different groups of blood donors. JAMA 1989:262:3452–3454.

Suggested Reading

Cumming PD, Wallace EL, Schorr JB, et al. Exposure of patients to human immunodeficiency virus through the transfusion of blood components that test antibody negative. N Engl J Med 1989;321:941–946.

Leslie SD, Toy P. Laboratory hemostatic abnormalities in massively transfused patients given red blood cells and crystalloid. Am J Clin Pathol 1991;96:770–773.

Morduchowicz G, Pitlik SD, Huminer D, et al. Transfusion reactions due to bacterial contamination of blood and blood products. Rev Infect Dis 1991;13:307–314.

Parkman R, Mosier D, Umansky I, et al. Graft versus host disease after intrauterine exchange transfusion for hemolytic disease of the newborn. N Engl J Med 1974;290:359–363.

Rossi EC, Simon TL, Moss GS, eds. Principles of transfusion medicine. Baltimore: Williams & Wilkins, 1991.

Sacks DA, Koppes RH. Blood transfusion and Jehovah's Witnesses: medical and legal issues in obstetrics and gynecology. Am J Obstet Gynecol 1986;154:483–486.

Summary of National Institutes of Health consensus development statement on perioperative red cell transfusion. Am J Obstet Gynecol 1989;160:278.

Turgeon ML. Fundamentals of immunohematology: theory and technique. Philadelphia: Lea & Febiger, 1989.

BLOOD TRANSFUSION, AUTOLOGOUS

Specimen Collection: Advise patients to avoid alcohol for 12 hours before the procedure and to increase their fluid intake.

Autologous donation may not be allowed if there is a possibility of bacteremia. This usually includes recent dental work.

Certain heart conditions may preclude autologous donation.

Usually the predonation hematocrit needs to be 34% or higher. Donations are usually given at weekly intervals or at most every 72 hours. Autologous donation is not performed < 72 hours before surgery.

Iron replacement needs to be provided to the patient (pre- and postdonation).

The blood can usually be stored under refrigeration for 35 days. If freezing of the blood is performed, it needs to be done within 5 days of the collection.

Clinical Correlation: The use of autologous transfusions avoids the problems of transmission of infection and transfusion reactions. A small risk of bacterial contamination of the specimen is similar to other blood donations.

Autologous donation is especially important for those patients with rare blood types or antibodies that limits their compatibility to a small number of donors.

Principle use for Ob/Gyn is donation before scheduled major gynecologic surgery.

Autologous blood donation has been clinically investigated during pregnancy for planned repeat cesarean section, grand multiparity, multiple gestation, placenta previa, and rare blood type. Early studies showed relative safety for donation, but there is still concern over possible effects on the fetus. Most studies indicate a low overall transfusion rate when evaluating all pregnancies. Of higher risk pregnancies, placenta previa patients require more transfusions. Further studies are needed to clearly define the conditions that would most benefit from autologous donation during pregnancy.

Suggested Reading

Andres RL, Piacquadio KM, Resnik R. A reappraisal of the need for autologous blood donation in the obstetric patient. Am J Obstet Gynecol 1990;163: 1551–1553.

Goodnough LT, Rudnick S, Price TH, et al. Increased preoperative collection of autologous blood with recombinant human erythropoietin therapy. N Engl J Med 1989;321:1163–1168.

Herbert WN, Owen HG, Collins ML. Autologous blood storage in obstetrics. Obstet Gynecol 1988;72:166–170.

Kruskall MS. Controversies in transfusion medicine. The safety and utility of autologous donations by pregnant patients: pro. Transfusion 1990;30:168–171.

Kruskall MS, Leonard S, Klapholz H. Autologous blood donation during pregnancy: analysis of safety and blood use. Obstet Gynecol 1987;70:938–941.

Simon TL. Postpartum blood requirements: should autologous donation programs be considered? JAMA 1988;259:2021.

BLOOD UREA NITROGEN (BUN)

Specimen Collection: Serum

Reference Range: 8–20 mg/dL (2.8–7.1 mmol/L) gradual increase with age

Clinical Correlation: The major product of protein catabolism is urea. It is synthesized in the liver and excreted in the kidneys with some degree of tubular reabsorption.

BUN determination is used primarily for evaluation of renal status. This test should be used in conjunction with creatinine measurement. As a test for renal function, BUN has the limitations in that it is also altered by protein intake, state of hydration, infections, protein catabolism, and urinary flow rates.

BUN decreases in the first trimester and remains lower than normal during pregnancy. Low levels may also be found in patients with low protein diets.

Prerenal azotemia (ie, dehydration, blood loss) will demonstrate an increased BUN/creatinine ratio (> 15:1).

Borrelia burgdorferi

Organism: Spirochete, transmitted by a tick (*Ixodes dammini*)
Other ticks suspected as vectors—*Ixodes pacificus, Amblyoma america*

Specimen Collection: Serum, cerebrospinal fluid (CSF), biopsy

Identification: Direct culture of organism is difficult.
Serology can be performed on serum and CSF specimens (IgG and IgM).

Serologic tests may be negative early in the disease course (rash stage) and seroconversion may not occur if antibiotics are taken. False positive serologic tests can also occur (infectious mononucleosis, positive rheumatoid factor, lupus, and other spirochetal disease). Western blot testing may add additional laboratory information but can be equivocal early in the course of the disease. Antibody capture techniques and use of a flagellar antigen in testing methods have improved the laboratory diagnosis, but standardization problems are still to be resolved.

Clinical Correlation: *B burgdorferi* is the causative organism for Lyme disease.

Concern about maternal-fetal transmission has been reported (1,2). Further studies are ongoing to determine if the organism has teratogenic potential.

If Lyme disease is suspected in fetal loss, culture and tissue stains should be used in the placenta and fetal organs.

References

1. Schlesinger PA, Duray PH, Burke BA, et al. Maternal-fetal transmission of the Lyme disease spirochete, *Borrelia burgdorferi*. Ann Intern Med 1985;103:67–68.
2. Markowitz LE, Steere AC, Benach JL, Slade JD, Broome CV. Lyme disease during pregnancy. JAMA 1986;255:3394–3396.

Suggested Reading

Kaslow RA. Current perspective on Lyme borreliosis. JAMA 1992;267:1381–1383.
Rahn DW, Malawista SE. Lyme disease: recommendations for diagnosis and treatment. Ann Intern Med 1991;114:472–481.
Smith LG Jr, Pearlman M, Smith LG, Faro S. Lyme disease: a review with emphasis on the pregnant woman. Obstet Gynecol Surv 1991;46:125–130.

CA 125

Specimen Collection: Serum

Reference Range: < 35 units/mL (radioimmunoassay)

Clinical Correlation: CA 125 is a glycoprotein expressed by approximately 80% of nonmucinous ovarian neoplasms. The test is ordered in patients presenting with adnexal masses and used as a tumor marker for follow-up care. It is not recommended as a screening test.

CA 125 is elevated in other conditions disruptive of the peritoneum (infections, endometriosis). Studies have shown some test benefit in the diagnosis and treatment response in endometriosis.

Suggested Reading

Barbieri RL, Niloff JM, Bast RC Jr, Scaetzl E, Kistner RW, Knapp RC. Elevated serum concentrations of CA 125 in patients with advanced endometriosis. Fertil Steril 1986;45:630–634.

Bast RC, Clug TL, St. John E, et al. A radioimmunoassay using a monoclonal antibody to monitor the course of epithelial ovarian carcinoma. N Engl J Med 1983;309:169–171.

Jacobs IJ, Bast RC. The CA 125 tumor associated antigen; a review of the literature. Hum Reprod 1989; 4:1–12.

Pittaway DE. The use of serial CA 125 concentrations to monitor endometriosis in infertile women. Am J Obstet Gynecol 1990;163:1032–1035.

CALCIUM, SERUM AND URINE

Specimen Collection: Serum, (venous stasis can affect levels)
24-hour urine collection, (acidified to dissolve calcium salts)

Reference Range:

Serum	8.4–10.2 mg/dL (2.10–2.55 mmol/L)
Serum, ionized	4.0–4.8 mg/dL (1.0–1.2 mmol/L)
Urine	100–250 mg/d (2.5–6.2 mmol/d) in nonpregnant individuals
Urine	350–650 mg/d (8.8–16.3 mmol/d) in pregnant individuals

Clinical Correlation:

Serum

Calcium, the most abundant mineral in the body, is important for skeletal development, blood coagulation, neuromuscular conduction, and enzyme activity. Calcium blood levels are affected by interactions of parathyroid hormone, vitamin D, calcitonin, and steroids. 50% of serum calcium is free or ionized, 45% is bound to plasma proteins, primarily albumin, and 5% is complexed with anions.

Decreased calcium levels detected in pregnancy are for the most part secondary to decreased plasma proteins (albumin). Ionized calcium shows little change from nonpregnant levels.

Small cell cancer of the ovary is associated with hypercalcemia. This rare tumor is in the sex-cord stromal group. It has been seen more often in younger women and has a poor prognosis.

A massive blood transfusion with citrated blood can lower calcium.

Serum calcium is normal in primary osteoporosis, but elevated with hyperparathyroidism.

Low levels may be present in acute pancreatitis. This is thought to be secondary to calcium sequestration in areas of fat necrosis.

Urine

Hypocalciuria has been used as a predictive test for preeclampsia (levels < 195 mg/d).

Causes for hypercalciuria may include hyperparathyroidism, metastatic bone disease, vitamin D intoxication, and Cushing's syndrome.

Suggested Reading

Taufield PA, Ales KL, Resnick LM, Druzin ML, Gertner JM, Laragh JH. Hypocalcuria in preeclampsia. N Engl J Med 1987;316:715.

Calymmatobacterium granulomatis

Organism: Nonmotile, non–spore-forming, encapsulated coccobacillus

Specimen Collection: Take biopsy or scraping from the base of the ulcerated lesion and prepare multiple touch prep slides (air dry). Gently prepare slides to avoid disrupting diagnostic cells.

Identification: Staining—Gram-negative (Giemsa or Wright staining is used to evaluate the tissue or scrape touch preps for Donovan bodies). Occasionally Donovan bodies can be identified with silver stains in histologic preparations.

The organism will also grow in chick embryo yolk sac and egg yolk slant preparations.

Clinical Correlation: This is the causative organism for granuloma inguinale. The clinical manifestations are ulcerating lesions in the genital and anal areas, labial swelling, and pseudobuboes, which represent subcutaneous granulation tissue.

Suggested Reading

Kellogg D, Majmudar B. Granuloma inguinale. In: Morse SA, Moreland AA, Thompson SE, eds. Atlas of sexually transmitted diseases. Philadelphia: JB Lippincott, 1990.

Candida SPECIES

Organism: Fungal organism (*Candida albicans, Candida glabrata,* and *Candida tropicalis*)

Specimen Collection: Vaginal swab of discharge, vulvar scrape. (A few drops of 10% to 15% KOH is added to the slide to allow for easier identification of the organism.)

Swab for culture (can use Culturette®), Sabouraud's media allow for the growth of the clinically important species.

Identification: Microscopic identification of yeast and pseudohyphae on wet smear preparations.

Pap smears and Gram stains will also identify organisms. *Candida* species are gram positive.

Culture methods

Clinical Correlation: *Candida* species play a significant role in vulvovaginitis with the production of thick curdy discharge and pruritic symptoms.

CD4 (T4-HELPER/INDUCER CELLS)

Specimen Collection: Heparin or EDTA

Reference Range: 32% to 50% of blood lymphocytes, 400–1600 cells/µL

Clinical Correlation: Decreased levels of CD4 cells are seen in HIV-positive patients with initial infection and then later when constitutional symptoms and opportunistic infections are present. Risk is high when CD4 is < 200/µL or a rapid decline has been noted. CD4 levels of < 200/µL now qualify as diagnostic of AIDS regardless of symptoms.

CD4 determinations are performed every 6 months for nonpregnant, HIV-positive individuals with counts > 600 cells/µL and every 3 months for counts of 200–600/µL. Counts < 200 cells/µL are associated with an increased risk of opportunistic infections. Some have recommended that HIV-positive pregnant patients have CD4 levels performed each trimester.

Suggested Reading

Sperling RS, Stratton P, members of the Obstetric-Gynecologic Working Group of the AIDS Clinical Trials Group of the National Institute of Allergy and Infectious Diseases. Treatment options for human immunodeficiency virus-infected pregnant women. Obstet Gynecol 1992;79:443–448.

Chlamydia trachomatis

Organism: Nonmotile bacteria with extra and intracellular stages in life cycle

Specimen Collection: If collecting a specimen for culture, use Dacron- or rayon-tipped plastic swabs.

Endocervical brush specimens are used for direct fluorescent testing. Smaller swabs for urethral specimens are provided in the kits.

If evaluating for lymphogranuloma venereum (LGV), draw acute and convalescent serum.

Identification: Cell culture (McCoy cell)
Enzyme immunoassay (Chlamydiazyme®)
Direct fluorescent antibody (Microtrak®)
DNA probe (GenProbe®)
Pap smear—Although lymphohistiocytic cell collections and metaplastic cell vacuoles containing small particles have been associated with chlamydia in some studies, both of these features on a Pap smear have suffered in terms of sensitivity and specificity. The 1991 modification of the Bethesda classification does not include chlamydia in the infection section.
LGV
Serology—The major use of serology in chlamydial infection is related to the diagnosis of LGV. Complement fixation values > 1:64 are considered positive. Because the test cross-reacts with all chlamydial infections, clinical correlation is needed.

McCoy cell culture may be positive.
Frei skin test is no longer performed.
A fourfold serologic titer increase is diagnostic.

Clinical Correlation: Testing for chlamydia may be performed in the following situations:

1. History of exposure
2. Suspicious vaginal discharge, cervicitis
3. Urethral syndrome
4. Routinely in prenatal exams
5. Suspicion of pelvic inflammatory disease
6. Nodal disease suspicious for LGV

The immunotypes associated with cervicitis, salpingitis, and urethritis are D, E, F, G, H, I, J, and K. The immunotypes of LGV are L_1, L_2, and L_3.

Suggested Reading

Barnes RC. Laboratory diagnosis of human chlamydial infections. Clin Microbiol Rev 1989;2:119–136.

Ehret JM, Judson FN. Genital chlamydia infections. Clin Lab Med 1989;9:481–500.

Graber DC, Williamson O, Pike J, et al. Detection of *Chlamydia trachomatis* infection in endocervical specimens using direct immunofluorescence. Obstet Gynecol 1985;66:727.

Tam MR, Stamm WE, Handsfield HH, et al. Culture independent diagnosis of *Chlamydia trachomatis* using monoclonal antibodies. N Engl J Med 1984; 310:1146.

Wentworth BB, Alexander ER. Isolation of *Chlamydia trachomatis* by use of 5-iodo-2-deoxyuridine treated cells. Appl Microbiol 1974;27:912.

CHOLESTEROL

Specimen Collection: Serum, nonfasting for total cholesterol

Fasting serum for lipid profile testing—fast for 12 hours, avoid dietary changes for preceding 3 weeks.

Venous stasis can increase cholesterol levels by 2% to 5%.

Reference Range:

Total cholesterol

Desirable	< 200 mg/dL (5.17 mmol/L)
Borderline	200–239 mg/dL (5.17–6.18 mmol/L)
High	> 240 mg/dL (6.2 mmol/L)

High-density lipoprotein (HDL) cholesterol
   35–65 mg/dL (0.9–1.7 mmol/L)

Low-density lipoprotein (LDL) cholesterol
   The level is usually calculated based on a formula using total cholesterol, HDL cholesterol, and triglycerides. The formula cannot be used if
the triglyceride level is > 400 mg/dL.

Desirable	< 130 mg/dL (3.4 mmol/L)
Borderline	130–159 mg/dL (3.4–4.1 mmol/L)
High risk	> 160 mg/dL (4.1 mmol/L)

Clinical Correlation: Cholesterol testing is used in health maintenance
care for all adults. Cardiovascular disease risk is associated with cholesterol levels. With normal levels, patients are evaluated at 5-year intervals.
Total cholesterol measurements are usually performed first. Fasting profiles that include HDL and LDL are performed secondarily if total cholesterol is elevated.

   Cholesterol levels are increased during pregnancy (about twofold elevation near term).

   Significant cholesterol elevation can occur in postmenopausal women
who are not taking replacement hormones.

   Hyperandrogenic patients should have cholesterol determinations made.

Clostridium difficile

Organism: Gram-positive anaerobe

Specimen Collection: Stool specimen for toxin assay, deliver immediately
to the laboratory. Refrigeration helps to prevent toxin deterioration.

Identification: Cytotoxin assay—The toxin in a bacteria-free stool ex-
tract will exert a cytopathic effect on certain cell culture lines. Results
reported as positive or negative. Latex agglutination methods, though
quicker, lack sensitivity.

Clinical Correlation: Colitis can occur in association with overgrowth of
toxin producing strains of *C difficile* secondary to antibiotic use. Symptoms include diarrhea, abdominal pain, and fever. A low threshold should
be maintained by the clinician for this problem. Cudmore and colleagues
(1) have also reported this complication in association with cytotoxic
chemotherapy.

Reference

1. Cudmore MA, Silva J, Fekety R, Liepman MK, Kim K. *Clostridium difficile* colitis: association with cancer chemotherapy. Arch Intern Med 1982;142: 333–335.

Suggested Reading

Lyerly DM, Krivan HC, Wilkins TD. *Clostridium difficile:* its disease and toxins. Clin Microbiol Rev 1988;1:1–18.
Styrt B, Gorbach SL. Recent developments in the understanding of the pathogenesis and treatment of anaerobic infections. N Engl J Med 1989;321:240.

Clostridium perfringens

Organism: Gram-positive anaerobe

Specimen Collection: May be able to obtain fluid from skin bullae
Blood for culture

Identification: Gram stain—gram-positive rods
Culture—anaerobic culture may be difficult from wound, blood culture

Clinical Correlation: Along with other clostridial species, this organism has been associated with myonecrosis (gas gangrene) and enteritis.

In clostridial myonecrosis, *α toxin* is one of the lethal exotoxins leading to cell destruction.

Diagnosis relies on palpation of crepitus, radiologic identification of gas, skin appearance, and incisional evidence.

Laboratory assessment for exotoxin-induced hemolytic anemia is important if clostridial infection is documented.

Blood cultures from a small percentage of patients with septic abortion are positive for *C perfringens*.

COMPLEMENT

Specimen Collection: Serum

Reference Range:

Total complement CH_{50}	50–200 units
C3	100–200 mg/dL (1.0–2.0 g/L)
C4	10–70 mg/dL (0.1–0.7 g/L)

Clinical Correlation: During pregnancy complement levels may be elevated.

Complement measurements have been recommended in the monitoring of pregnant patients with lupus. Falling or low levels tend to indicate disease activation, but the clinician should be aware that the levels do not always correspond to clinical manifestations. Other laboratory parameters that are frequently monitored for the pregnant patient with lupus include CBC, retic count, platelets, liver enzymes, urinalysis, and creatinine. (Evaluation for hemolysis, leukopenia, thrombocytopenia, hepatic, and renal dysfunction)

Depressed complement levels may also be found in the rarely occurring glomerulonephritis in pregnancy.

COMPLETE BLOOD COUNT (CBC)

Specimen Collection: EDTA

Reference Range:

Erythrocyte	biconcave, 6.7–7.8 µm in diameter, zone of central pallor	
Hemoglobin (Hgb)	12–16 g/dL	(120–160 g/L)
Pregnancy	Decreased by 1.5–2.0 g/dL	
Hematocrit (Hct)	37–47%	(0.37–0.47)
Pregnancy	Decreased by 4–6%	
Red blood cell count	$4.2–5.4 \times 10^6/\mu L$	$(4.2–5.4 \times 10^{12}/L)$
Pregnancy	Decreased by $0.8 \times 10^6/\mu L$	
Mean cell volume (MCV)	81–99 µm³	(81–99 fL)
Mean cell hemoglobin (MCH)	27–31 pg	(27–31 pg)
Mean cell hemoglobin concentration (MCHC)	33–37 g/dL	(330–370 g/L)
White blood cell count	$4.8–10.8 \times 10^3/uL$	$(4.8–10.8 \times 10^9/L)$
White blood cell differential		
segs	53–79%	
bands	1–10%	
eos	0–4%	
lymph	13–46%	
monos	3–9%	
basos	0–1%	

Clinical Correlation: The CBC (or its components) are frequently used by Ob-Gyn clinicians in numerous conditions including:

1. Diagnosis and further assessment of anemia (microcytic vs macrocytic)
2. Assessment of white blood cell count and differential in infections, diseases of the immune system, patients receiving chemotherapy
3. Monitoring of patients receiving blood component therapy
4. Health maintenance screening

During pregnancy increased blood volume is caused by increases in both plasma and erythrocytes. There is a larger increase in plasma volume. As a result, the CBC shows a slight decrease in erythrocytes, hematocrit, and hemoglobin in normal pregnancy.

During pregnancy the white blood cell count averages $7.0 \times 10^3/\mu L$ in the first trimester and $10.0 \times 10^3/\mu L$ in the third trimester. A further increase to $20.0 \times 10^3/\mu L$ and above can occur with labor.

Anemia in pregnancy has been defined by the Centers for Disease Control and Prevention (1) as hemoglobin values < 11 g/dL in the first and third trimesters and < 10.5 g/dL in the second trimester. Anemia laboratory work-ups are similar to those in nonpregnant patients, incorporating red cell indices, peripheral smear, ferritin, folate, B_{12}, etc. Whenever an anemia evaluation is performed, the clinician should not overlook evidence of multifactorial causation. This may be detected through patient history or suspected if laboratory findings do not fit just one picture.

Red cell morphology is helpful in identifying certain disease processes.

Hypochromia and microcytosis (< 6.5 µm)	Iron deficiency anemia Thalassemia
Leptocytes	Target cells, seen in association with thalassemia
Macrocytosis ($9–12$ µm)	Folic acid deficiency B_{12} deficiency
Poikilocytosis	Sickle cell disease Hemolysis
Drepanocytes	Sickle cells
Schistocytosis	Hemolysis
Spherocytosis	Hereditary spherocytosis Autoimmune hemolytic anemia

Pregnant women with systemic lupus, inflammatory bowel disease, rheumatoid arthritis, and chronic renal disease may manifest anemia of chronic disease that is refractory to treatment.

Hemolytic anemia encountered in Ob/Gyn

1. Drug induced (cephalosporins, penicillin, methyldopa erythromycin, acetaminophen, etc)
2. In some cases of preeclampsia-eclampsia
3. Secondary to exotoxin of *Clostridium perfringens*

Reference

1. Centers for Disease Control. CDC criteria for anemia in children and childbearing women. MMWR 1989;38:400.

CORTISOL, SERUM AND URINARY FREE

Specimen Collection: Serum

24-hour urine collection, refrigeration, preservative to keep specimen at 4.0–4.5 pH.

Reference Range

Serum
AM—5–25 µg/dL (138–690 nmol/L)
PM—3–13 µg/dL (83–359 nmol/L)
Dexamethasone suppression
    1 mg overnight (ingestion of 1 mg at 2300, serum cortisol at 0800)—
    > 5 µg/dL = nonsuppressed
Urinary Free Cortisol
24–108 µg/d (60–300 nmol/d)

Clinical Correlation: The Ob/Gyn clinician may be the first to encounter the rare patient with spontaneously occurring Cushing's syndrome, especially in relationship to complaints of hirsutism and menstrual disorders. Initial screening tests include overnight dexamethasone suppression and 24-hour urinary free cortisol. Most patients with equivocal or positive testing will be referred to endocrinologists for additional testing (high-dose suppression, computed tomography scans, corticotropin, etc).

C-REACTIVE PROTEIN

Specimen Collection: Serum

Reference Range: Normally < 8 mg/L

Clinical Correlation: C-reactive protein, which is synthesized in the liver, was the first acute phase reactant to be discovered. This test is a fairly sensitive but not a very specific indicator of infection.

In obstetrics this test has been evaluated in the prediction of intra-amniotic infection in women with premature rupture of the membranes (1,2). A slight elevation occurs in normal pregnancies (3). Serial measurements > 20 mg/L and very high levels appear to be more helpful in assessing for infection (2). C-reactive protein should be used in conjunction with other clinical and laboratory assessments in the patient with premature rupture of the membranes.

In gynecology, this test is used for monitoring results of treatment for pelvic inflammatory disease (4,5).

References

1. Ismail MA, Zinaman MJ, Lowensohn RI, Moawad AH. The significance of C-reactive protein levels in women with premature rupture of membranes. Am J Obstet Gynecol 1985;151:541–544.
2. Fisk NM, Fysh J, Child AG, Gatenby PA, Jeffery H, Bradfield AH. Is C-reactive protein really useful in preterm premature rupture of the membranes? Br J Obstet Gynaecol 1987;94:1159–1164.
3. Watts DH, Krohn MA, Wener MH, Eschenbach DA. C-reactive protein in normal pregnancy. Obstet Gynecol 1991;77:176–180.
4. Lehtinen M, Laine S, Heinonen PK. Serum C-reactive protein determination in acute pelvic inflammatory disease. Am J Obstet Gynecol 1986;154:158–159.
5. Teisala K, Heinonen PK. C-reactive protein in assessing antimicrobial treatment of acute pelvic inflammatory disease. J Reprod Med 1990;35:955.

CREATININE, SERUM

Specimen Collection: Serum
Interference may occur with noncreatinine chromogens.

Reference Range: 0.6–1.2 mg/dL (53–106 µmol/L)
Pregnancy 0.4–0.8 mg/dL (35–71 µmol/L)

Clinical Correlation: Serum creatinine is slightly reduced in pregnancy secondary to increased glomerular filtration. Careful evaluation for renal disease is needed for creatinine levels $> 0.9–1.0$ mg/dL in pregnancy.

A reduction in glomerular filtration can occur in acute pyelonephritis in pregnancy and creatinine determinations should be performed.

Creatinine levels and renal insufficiency:

$$1.4–2.5 \text{ mg/dL} \quad \text{moderate}$$
$$> 2.5 \text{ mg/dL} \quad \text{severe}$$

Laboratory creatinine determinations can be affected by drugs and metabolic conditions (ie, cephalosporins, trimethoprim, cimetidine, ketones, glucose)

CREATININE CLEARANCE

Specimen Collection: Timed urine collection (2, 6, 12, 24 hours)
Serum collection for measurement of creatinine obtained during urine collection period.

Reference Range: 75–115 mL/min/1.73 m² (1.25–1.92 mL/s/1.73 m²)
In pregnancy the creatinine clearance can increase 40%.

Clinical Correlation: Creatinine clearance represents the volume of blood that can be cleared of creatinine in one minute. This test is used to evaluate glomerular filtration rate.

This test is frequently performed in pregnant patients with renal disease and also to evaluate the insulin-dependent diabetic patient's renal function during pregnancy.

A reduced clearance may be seen in association with shock, intrinsic renal disease, and urinary tract obstruction.

Glomerular filtration rates and renal plasma flow both increase in pregnancy. Creatinine clearance is usually about 40% greater than the nongravid patient.

With progressive renal failure and high serum creatinine, tubular secretion of creatinine can lead to creatinine clearance overestimation.

Cryptococcus neoformans

Organism: Yeast organism

Specimen Collection: Sputum, blood, skin lesion, cerebrospinal fluid (CSF) for culture
Serum and CSF for serology

Identification: Culture
CSF India ink preparation, microscopic evaluation of other sites
Latex agglutination

Clinical Correlation: See Chapter 6 on fungal and parasitic infections.

CYTOMEGALOVIRUS (CMV)

Organism: Double-stranded DNA virus

Specimen Collection: Culture—*urine* (midstream early morning specimen in sterile container), *blood* (10–15 mL mixed with 500 units preservative-free heparin), *saliva/throat* (swab-viral transport medium), *cervical secretion* (swab-viral transport medium)
Serology—red top tube

Results: Culture results are obtained anywhere from 1–14 days depending on method. Shell vial method can give results within 24 hours.

Primary infection diagnosis by newly appearing IgM or fourfold rise in IgG in previously seronegative patient. It should be noted that reactivation can also induce a CMV-IgM response. False positives have been seen (with + rheumatoid factor, acute Epstein-Barr virus infection).

Clinical Correlation: CMV antibodies are found in 60% to 90% of adults in the United States.

Viral cultures show active infection but cannot differentiate between primary infection, reactivation of latent infection, or reinfection.

Risk of severe congenital infection is greater when the maternal infection is primary, but laboratory studies are poor predictors of risk.

High CMV titers may be found in AIDS patients.

DEHYDROEPIANDROSTERONE SULFATE (DHEAS)

Specimen Collection: Serum

Reference Range: Decreasing levels noted with age:

20–29	0.7–4.6 µg/mL
30–39	0.5–4.1 µg/mL
40–49	0.4–3.4 µg/mL
50–59	0.3–2.7 µg/mL
60–69	0.2–1.7 µg/mL

Clinical Correlation: As noted in Chapter 20 on hyperandrogenism, DHEAS measurement plays a limited role in the evaluation of hirsute women.

DIGITOXIN, DIGOXIN

Specimen Collection: Serum, plasma

Therapeutic Range: Digitoxin—15–30 ng/mL (19.2–38.5 nmol/L)
Digoxin—1–2 ng/mL (1.3–2.6 nmol/L)

Clinical Correlation: Treatment with digitalis during pregnancy may be related to either maternal or fetal heart problems (ie, peripartum cardiomyopathy, fetal supraventricular tachycardia).

Care needs to be taken to evaluate renal status, metabolic disorders, and other medications that may contribute to digitalis toxicity. Carefully assess timing of specimen collection if an elevated level is found.

The production of a digoxin-like substance (1) during pregnancy may falsely elevate clinical laboratory measurements.

Reference

1. Graves SW, Valdes JR, Brown BA, et al. Endogenous digoxin-substance in human pregnancies. J Clin Endocrinol Metab 1984;58:748–751.

DISATURATED PHOSPHATIDYLCHOLINE

Specimen Collection: Amniotic fluid, test may be altered by volume effects (oligohydramnios and polyhydramnios)

Reference Range: Levels of 500 µg/dL correlate with maturity (check with laboratory because values may vary with methodology).

Clinical Correlation: This is the major component of surfactant. Some methods are more complicated than lecithin/sphingomyelin ratio and it is not clear that this test offers any significant advantages.

Suggested Reading

Nugent CE, Ayers JW, Menon KM. Comparison of amniotic fluid disaturated phosphatidylcholine and the lecithin-sphingomyelin ratio in the prediction of fetal lung maturity. Obstet Gynecol 1986;68:541–545.

ELECTROLYTES

Specimen Collection: Serum

Reference Range

Chloride	98–109 mEq/L (98–109 mmol/L)
Sodium	137–145 mEq/L (137–145 mmol/L)
Potassium	3.5–5.0 mEq/L (3.5–5.0 mmol/L)
Bicarbonate	21–28 mmol/L (21–28 mmol/L)

Clinical Correlation: Electrolyte determinations are important for any patient requiring fluid maintenance or on medications that alter the normal levels.

Potassium ($\downarrow$ 0.2–0.3 mEq/L) and sodium ($\downarrow$ 2–4 mEq/L) levels are slightly decreased in pregnancy.

Hypokalemia most often encountered by the clinician in Ob/Gyn:

Secondary to diuretic therapy
Secondary to vomiting, nasogastric suctioning, intestinal fluid loss
Secondary to β-mimetic tocolytic therapy

Hyperkalemia may be encountered in women with renal failure or in infants with congenital adrenal hyperplasia.

Severe hyponatremia can occur as a complication of oxytocin infusion administered in large volumes of electrolyte-free dextrose solutions. Hyponatremia will also result when body salt losses are replaced with these solutions alone.

Hypernatremia is rare. It can result from diabetes insipidus or excess salt loading.

Suggested Reading

Abdul-Karim R, Assali NS. Renal function in human pregnancy: V. Effects of oxytocin on renal hemodynamics and water and electrolyte excretion. J Lab Clin Med 1961;57:522.

Young D, Toofanian A, Leveno K. Potassium and glucose concentrations without treatment during ritodrine tocolysis. Am J Obstet Gynecol 1983;145:105.

Entamoeba histolytica

Organism: Protozoan

Specimen Collection: Stool, rectal biopsy, serum

Identification: Stool identification can be very difficult (false negatives and positives); supravital staining can be very helpful.
    Microscopic diagnosis from biopsy
    Serology—indirect hemagglutination

Clinical Correlation: See Chapter 6 on fungal and parasitic infections.

Enterobius vermicularis

Organism: Intestinal nematode

Specimen Collection: Swab from perineum or cellulose tape test
    Care in handling—pinworm eggs are infectious

Identification: Ova identification—elongate in shape, approximately 50 microns in length
    Rare identification has been made on Pap smear.

Clinical Correlation: Should be considered as a cause for vaginitis, especially in the prepubertal female.
    Migration of the organism to unusual sites has included the uterus, fallopian tubes, and peritoneal cavity. A granulomatous tissue response may occur.

ERYTHROCYTE SEDIMENTATION RATE (ESR)

Specimen Collection: EDTA, sodium citrate, or sodium oxalate tubes may be used, depending on laboratory methodology. Completely fill tube, mix.

Reference Range: Normally < 20 mm/h, range increases with age (0–35 mm/h, at age > 55 years).

Clinical Correlation: The ESR measures the time it takes for blood to settle in a vertical tube. Factors that influence settling rate include red cell volume, surface charge, aggregation, and plasma proteins.

This nonspecific test is elevated in a number of conditions including pregnancy, inflammations, autoimmune conditions, neoplastic conditions, and anemia. The test may also be used serially to evaluate improvement of a condition (pelvic infection response to antimicrobials).

ESTRADIOL (E_2)

Specimen Collection: Serum

Reference Range

Prepubertal	< 20 pg/mL
Follicular	25–90 pg/mL
Midcycle	100–500 pg/mL
Luteal	100–280 pg/mL
Postmenopausal	5–25 pg/mL

Clinical Correlation: E_2 measurements are performed in patients undergoing ovarian stimulation with human menopausal gonadotropin. Attempts are made to attain levels close to 1000 pg/mL. Levels > 1500–2000 pg/mL put the patient at risk for developing ovarian hyperstimulation syndrome. E_2 levels in this setting are used in conjunction with sonographic monitoring of follicular development.

E_2 is one of the laboratory tests used in the evaluation of precocious puberty. It is also used to monitor treatment of this condition.

As noted in Chapter 24 on assisted reproduction, basal E_2 measurements may help to predict outcome of in vitro fertilization.

Suggested Reading

Ho Yuen B, Sy L, Cannon W. Regulation of ovarian and luteal function during treatment with exogenous gonadotropins in anovulatory infertility. Am J Obstet Gynecol 1981;140:629–635.

Pride SM, James C, Ho Yuen B. The ovarian hyperstimulation syndrome. Semin Reprod Endocrinol 1990;8:247.

ESTRIOL, UNCONJUGATED

Specimen Collection: Serum

Clinical Correlation: Combined with α-fetoprotein and human chorionic gonadotropin in the triple screen to provide risk estimates for Down syndrome. Affected pregnancies may manifest a low unconjugated estriol level (see Chapter 10 on genetics).

ESTROGEN/PROGESTERONE RECEPTOR ASSAY

Specimen Collection: One gram of tissue, quickly frozen in liquid nitrogen

Reference Range: Negative (binding capacity in femtomoles of labeled steroid bound per mg cytosol protein)

Clinical Correlation: Submission of tumor tissue from endometrial and ovarian cancers for estrogen receptors may be of clinical benefit (see Chapter 26 on tumor markers).

FECAL OCCULT BLOOD TESTING

Specimen Collection: Stool specimen (many clinicians perform in the office). Three specimens collected by patient may improve testing. Recommended that patient send in the cards soon after performing the test. Avoiding meat, peroxidase-rich vegetables, and gastric irritants helps to prevent false positive results.

Clinical Correlation: See Chapter 1 on health maintenance.

FERN TEST

Specimen Collection: Vaginal fluid (avoid the cervix because cervical mucus can also show a coarse ferning pattern)

Clinical Correlation: This test is used for evaluation of ruptured membranes. It is unaffected by meconium and pH (1).

Ferning can still be detected in amniotic fluid contaminated with blood, but may have an altered "skeletonized" pattern (2).

References

1. Reece EA, Chervenak F, Moya F, et al. Amniotic fluid arborization: effect of blood, meconium, and pH alterations. Obstet Gynecol 1984;64:248–250.
2. Rosemond RL, Lombardi SJ, Boehm FH. Ferning of amniotic fluid contaminated with blood. Obstet Gynecol 1990;75:338–340.

FERRITIN

Specimen Collection: Serum

Reference Range: 12–150 ng/mL (12–150 µg/L)

Ferritin levels increase slightly in the first trimester and then decrease on into the third trimester.

Clinical Correlation: Ferritin generally correlates with storage iron. Levels < 12 ng/mL indicate absent iron stores. Normal to high ferritin levels are found in the anemia of chronic disease.

If ferritin is being used to monitor iron therapy, the treatment is continued until the ferritin is in the 50 ng/mL range.

A normal ferritin level does not always exclude iron deficiency because it is an acute phase reactant and can be elevated in the presence of inflammation.

Suggested Reading

Jacobs A, Worwood M. Ferritin in serum. Clinical and biochemical implications. N Engl J Med 1975;292:951–956.

FETAL BLOOD STUDIES

Specimen Collection: Cord blood aspiration (or intrahepatic venous sampling) under sonographic guidance. Mean corpuscular volume and Kleihauer-Betke testing are used to ensure that the specimen is fetal in origin.

Reference Range: The reader is directed to the Daffos reference (1) for normal laboratory levels.

Clinical Correlation: Fetal blood studies may be used in the following situations:

1. Chromosomal analysis
    a. Late second trimester evaluation
    b. Evaluation of polyhydramnios, oligohydramnios, intrauterine growth rate, fetal anomalies
    c. Distinguishing true mosaicism
2. Infectious disease
    a. Toxoplasmosis
    b. Cytomegalovirus
    c. Rubella
    d. Parvovirus B19
    e. Varicella
3. Hematologic disorders
    a. Isoimmunization
    b. Thrombocytopenias (immune, isoimmune)
    c. Hemophilia
    d. Hemoglobinopathies
4. Immunodeficiency disorders

Reference

1. Daffos F. Fetal blood sampling. In: Harrison WR, Golbus MS, Filly RA, eds. The unborn patient, 2d ed. Philadelphia: WB Saunders, 1991:79.

Suggested Reading

Cuthbertson G, Weiner CO, Giller RH, Grose C. Prenatal diagnosis of second trimester congenital varicella syndrome by virus-specific IgM. J Pediatr 1987; 111:592–595.

Daffos F, Capella-Pavlovsky M, Forestier F. Fetal blood sampling during pregnancy with the use of a needle guided by ultrasound: a study of 606 consecutive cases. Am J Obstet Gynecol 1985;153:655–660.

Daffos F, Forestier F, Capella-Pavlovsky M, et al. Prenatal management of 746 pregnancies at risk for congenital toxoplasmosis. N Engl J Med 1988;318:271–275.

Daffos F, Forestier F, Grangeot-Keros L, et al. Prenatal diagnosis of congenital rubella. Lancet 1984;ii:1

Ludomirski A, Weiner S. Percutaneous fetal umbilical blood sampling. Clin Obstet Gynecol 1988;31:19–26.

Lynch L, Daffos F, Emanuel D, et al. Prenatal diagnosis of fetal cytomegalovirus infection. Am J Obstet Gynecol 1991;165:714–718.

Meizner I, Glezerman M. Cordocentesis in the evaluation of the growth-retarded fetus. Clin Obstet Gynecol 1992;35:126–137.

Nicolaides KH. Cordocentesis. Clin Obstet Gynecol 1988;31:123–135.

Peters MT, Nicolaides KH. Cordocentesis for the diagnosis and treatment of human fetal parvovirus infection. Obstet Gynecol 1990;75:501–504.

Wax JR, Blakemore KJ. What can be learned from cordocentesis? Clin Lab Med 1992;12:503–521.

FIBRIN DEGRADATION PRODUCTS

Specimen Collection: Tube containing thrombin and protease inhibitor

Reference Range: Normally < 10 µg/mL

Clinical Correlation: High levels are found in patients with consumptive coagulopathy (which arises in Ob-Gyn patients with placental abruption, fetal demise, bacterial toxins, and neoplasms).

Elevated levels are only rarely found in pregnancy-induced hypertension that is not associated with placental abruption.

FIBRINOGEN

Specimen Collection: Sodium citrate

Reference Range: 200–400 mg/dL

Pregnancy change—increased by 50% by end of the second trimester secondary to estrogen-stimulated production by the liver.

Clinical Correlation: Critical range—< 100 mg/dL

Used in evaluation of consumptive coagulopathy and in patients requiring massive blood transfusions.

Fibrinogen is an acute phase reactant and is elevated in inflammatory conditions.

FIBRONECTIN

Specimen Collection: Plasma, citrate

Reference range: 200–400 mg/dL

Clinical Correlation: Fibronectin is a glycoprotein that has been found to be elevated in women with preeclampsia. It may be detected before clinical manifestations of the disease (see Chapter 2 on hypertension).

Studies have also looked at fetal fibronectin as a marker for ruptured membranes and predictor of impending labor.

Suggested Reading

Ballegeer V, Spitz B, Kieckens L, Moreau H, Van Assche A, Collen D. Predictive value of increased plasma levels of fibronectin in gestational hypertension. Am J Obstet Gynecol 1989;161:432–436.

Brubaker DB, Ross MG, Marinoff D. The function of elevated plasma fibronectin in preeclampsia. Am J Obstet Gynecol 1992; 166:526–531.

Eriksen NL, Parisi VM, Daoust S, Flamm B, Garite TJ, Cox SM. Fetal fibronectin: a method for detecting the presence of amniotic fluid. Obstet Gynecol 1992;80: 451–454.

Lazarchick J, Stubbs TM, Romein L, Van Dorsten JP, Loadholt CB. Predictive value of fibronectin levels in normotensive gravid women destined to become preeclamptic. Am J Obstet Gynecol 1986;154:1050–1052.

Lockwood CJ, Peters JH. Increased plasma levels of ED1+ cellular fibronectin precede the clinical signs of preeclampsia. Am J Obstet Gynecol 1990;162: 358–362.

Lockwood CJ, Senyei AE, Dische MR, et al. Fetal fibronectin in cervical and vaginal secretions as a predictor of preterm delivery. N Engl J Med 1991;325: 669–674.

FOAM STABILITY INDEX (LUMADEX-FSI)

Specimen Collection: Amniotic fluid (blood and meconium affects the results)

Reference Range: A level of 47 or above correlates with maturity.

Clinical Correlation: This test is based on the Shake test but comes in a kit with predispensed volumes of ethanol.

Suggested Reading

Lipshitz J, Anderson GD, Whybrew WD. Accelerated pulmonary maturity as measured by the Lumadex foam stability index test. Obstet Gynecol 1983; 62:31–36.

Sher G, Statland GE. Assessment of fetal pulmonary maturity by the Lumadex foam stability index test. Obstet Gynecol 1983;61:444–449.

FOLIC ACID

Specimen Collection: Serum, fasting specimen preferred

Reference Range

Serum folate	3–15 µg/L (4–30 mmol/L)
Red cell folate	200–800 µg/L (400–1800 mmol/L)

Clinical Correlation: Folate deficiency can result from inadequate intake, drugs, impaired absorption, and increased utilization.

Folate levels are used (in conjunction with vitamin B_{12}) in the evaluation of macrocytic anemia.

Leukopenia and thrombocytopenia can accompany severe folate deficiency.

Red cell folate may be more reflective of tissue folate deficiency.

Morphologic evidence of folic acid deficiency includes macrocytosis and hypersegmentation of neutrophils.

FOLLICLE-STIMULATING HORMONE (FSH)

Specimen Collection: Serum

Reference Range

Women	
Prepubertal	< 10 mIU/mL (IU/L)
Follicular	5–20 mIU/mL (IU/L)
Midcycle	15–30 mIU/mL (IU/L)
Luteal	5–15 mIU/mL
Menopausal	40–100 mIU/mL
Men	< 15 mIU/mL

Clinical Correlation: FSH determinations serve a multitude of uses in Ob-Gyn. Clinical correlations are found in the following chapters:

1. Amenorrhea (Chapter 18)
2. Ovarian Failure (Chapter 19)
3. Hypothalamic Dysfunction (Chapter 21)
4. Female Fertility (Chapter 22)
5. Male Fertility (Chapter 23)
6. Assisted Reproductive Technology (Chapter 24)

There tends to be a gradual rise in FSH before menopause with an accompanying decrease in estradiol. Episodes of amenorrhea with elevated gonadotropins are sometimes followed by ovulatory cycles and normal levels of gonadotropins in the premenopausal time period.

FRUCTOSAMINE

Specimen Collection: Serum

Reference Range: 49–67 mg/dL (2.0–2.7 mmol/L) Reference range is lower in pregnancy.

Clinical Correlation: Evaluation of short-term control (3 weeks) in diabetes, as opposed to longer term control evaluation performed by measuring hemoglobin A_{1C}.
Useful in patients with conditions of increased red cell turnover.

Gardnerella vaginalis

Organism: Pleomorphic gram-variable bacillus, facultative

Clinical Correlation: See Chapter 13 on vulvovaginitis.

Giardia lamblia

Organism: Flagellated protozoan

Specimen Collection: Stool specimen (multiple specimens may be needed)
Intestinal aspirate, small bowel biopsy

Identification: Stool is examined for cysts and trophozoites; wet preparation of intestinal aspirate may reveal motile organisms. Histologic identification of small bowel biopsy may reveal organisms.

Clinical Correlation: See Chapter 6 on fungal and parasitic infections.

GLUCOSE

Specimen Collection: Sodium fluoride, serum

Reference Range: 60–115 mg/dL (3.3–6.4 mmol/L)

Clinical Correlation: See Chapter 3 (Diabetes in Pregnancy), Chapter 12 (Ambiguous Genitalia), and Chapter 25 (Oral Contraceptives).

GLYCOHEMOGLOBIN

Specimen Collection: Type of collection tube depends on methodology

Reference Range

HemoglobinA_{1C} 3.6–4.9% by high-performance liquid chromatography (HPLC)
Hemoglobin A_1 5.1–7.8% by HPLC

Clinical Correlation: Glycosylated hemoglobin is a test of long-term glucose control that reflects glycemia over 2–3 months. Hemoglobin A_1 consists of three components (A_{1a}, A_{1b}, and A_{1c}) of which A_{1c} is the most abundant.

GRAM STAIN

Methodology

1. Air dry thin smear
2. Alcohol fixation on slide warmer for 10 minutes
3. Crystal violet stain × 10–30 seconds, rinse with distilled water
4. Gram's iodine × 20–60 seconds, rinse with distilled water
5. Decolorize with acetone alcohol until violet color washes off (about 10 seconds)
6. Safranin stain × 30 seconds, dry, microscopic examination by oil

Results—Gram positive, dark blue; Gram negative, pink-red

Clinical Correlation: Gram-positive cocci include *Peptostreptococcus, Peptococcus, Streptococci,* and *Staphylococci.*

Gram-positive rods include corynebacteria, listeria, clostridia, and *Actinomyces*

Gram-negative cocci include *Neisseria gonorrhoeae*

Gram-negative rods include *Escherichia coli, Proteus, Klebsiella, Enterobacter Gardnerella, Pseudomonas,* and *Bacteroides* species

Suggested Reading

Provine H, Gardner P. The gram stained smear and its interpretation. Hosp Pract 1974;9:85–91.

Haemophilus ducreyi

Organism: Small gram-negative nonmotile rod, streptobacillary chains

Specimen Collection: Cotton or calcium alginate swab of ulcer base for Gram stain and culture. Some advise direct plating for culture at the time of collection. Call the laboratory ahead of time for their protocol.

Identification: Gram stain
Culture—very fastidious organism
Other methods include dot immunobinding assay, enzyme-linked immunosorbent assay

Clinical Correlation: *H ducreyi* is the causative organism for chanchroid. Most clinicians will only rarely be ordering tests for this organism and proper coordination with microbiology laboratory is important.

HEMIZONA ASSAY

Clinical Correlation: See Chapter 23 on male fertility.

HEMOGLOBIN (Hb) ELECTROPHORESIS

Specimen Collection: EDTA

Reference Range: Normally 95% to 98% Hb A, 2% to 3% Hb A_2, and < 1% Hb F. Hb S and C are normally absent.

Clinical Correlation: Determination of abnormal hemoglobin may be very complicated. Different electrophoretic techniques are used. Unstable variants may migrate along with others. Other confirmatory tests including molecular diagnostics may need to be used. In different cases the specimen may be sent to referral laboratories or the Centers for Disease Control and Prevention.

Hemoglobin electrophoresis is used in the diagnosis of hemoglobino-pathies and thalassemias, as well as part of the work-up for hemolytic anemia. Prenatal testing is performed for patients at risk.

Findings in disease:

	A	A_2	S	C	F
Sickle cell trait	50–60%	2–3%	40–45%		1%
Sickle cell disease	0	2–3%	85–95%		5–15%
SC disease	0	2–3%	45–50%	45–50%	1%

	A	A_2	F	Other
α-Thalassemia				
Homozygous	0	0	0	Hb Bart, H
Hb H	60–90%	1–2%	5–15%	Hb H (4–30%)
				Hb Bart (trace)
Minor	>95%	<3.5%	<2%	0

β-Thalassemia

Homozygous types—Different genotypes are possible, variable levels of Hb A_2, can have low to absent Hb A, increased Hb F at birth.
Heterozygous types—Different genotypes are possible, usually manifest increased Hb A_2 and Hb F with 80–95% Hb A.
Sickle β-thalassemia—Different genotypes, Hb A is low to absent, Hb S is 50% to 90%, increased levels of Hb A_2 and Hb F.

Additional laboratory testing of patients with sickle cell trait includes pe-riodic urinalysis and urine culture for evaluation of urinary tract infection.

Laboratory assessment of patients with sickle cell disease includes fre-quent evaluation of hemoglobin/hematocrit, hemoglobin electrophoresis, reticulocyte count, platelets, urinalysis, and urine cultures. Serum iron and ferritin should also be monitored. Similar laboratory management is used for SC and Sickle-β-thalassemia.

Hb H disease can manifest iron deficiency and the anemia may worsen during pregnancy.

Homozygous α-thalassemia is incapatible with life. It causes nonim-mune hydrops and death in utero.

α-Thalassemia minor manifests a mild to moderate hypochromic, mi-crocytic anemia. These women tolerate pregnancy well.

Homozygous β-thalassemia patients may have a life expectancy to the third decade. Rare successful pregnancies have been reported. Laboratory assessment of anemia and iron overloading are required.

Heterozygous forms of β-thalassemia usually do not cause great problems in pregnancy. Hemoglobin is usually in the 9–11 g/dL range with decreased mean corpuscular hemoglobin and mean corpuscular volume. Infections may worsen anemia. Care must be taken to avoid iron overloading.

HEPATITIS A VIRUS (HAV)

Organism: RNA enterovirus

Transmission/Incubation: Fecal and oral/2–6 weeks

Specimen Collection: Red top tube

Serology: Infection diagnosed with IgM or rise in IgG. Low titers of IgG consistent with previous infection.

Clinical Correlation: Hepatitis A does not cross the placenta; however, maternal infection in the last 6 weeks of pregnancy or postpartum carries the risk for exposure.

HEPATITIS B VIRUS (HBV)

Organism: Double-stranded DNA virus

Transmission/Incubation: Blood, saliva, semen, cervicovaginal secretions, placental transmission. Incubation is 5 weeks to 6 months.

Specimen Collection: Red top tube

Antigen Testing
Surface (HBsAg)
Elevated during incubation, early acute infection, recovery period, chronic hepatitis, and persistent carriers. Chronic carrier state is diagnosed with persistence of antigen for > 6 months.
e Antigen (HBeAg)
Appears with or shortly after HbsAg. Positivity for e antigen correlates with increased risk for transmission (including perinatal transmission). This test may also be used to evaluate patients on interferon therapy.

Antibody Testing: Antibody to surface antigen (anti-HBs) appears 2–6 weeks after the disappearance of HBsAg and peaks 2–8 weeks later with a decline to lower titers over many years. Rising titers are indicative of recovery. Titers are also elevated in persons vaccinated with HBV vaccine.

Antibody to e antigen (anti-HBe) indicates reduced infectivity.

IgM-specific antibody to hepatitis B core antigen (anti-HBc) indicates acute HBV with or without the presence of HBsAg.

Clinical Correlation: Hepatitis B testing is used in prenatal screens, evaluation of jaundice, evaluation of blood donor products, and in patients with elevated liver enzymes.

Hepatitis delta virus (HDV) is an incomplete RNA virus that may coinfect patients with HBV. IgG and IgM testing is available.

HEPATITIS C VIRUS (HCV)

Organism: Single-stranded RNA virus

Transmission/Incubation: Parenteral drug abuse, blood transfusion, sexual transmission, perinatal transmission

Serology: Anti-HCV testing has been hampered by false positive results and negativity in early stage disease. Immunoblot confirmation testing should be used.

Clinical Correlation: Testing is recommended for high-risk individuals. Perinatal transmission has been reported.

HERPES SIMPLEX VIRUS (HSV)

Organism: Double-stranded DNA virus, serotypes HSV-1 and HSV-2

Transmission/Incubation: Transmitted by saliva, eye secretions, genital secretions. Incubation is 5–10 days.

Specimen Collection

Culture—Aspirate or swab from lesions.

Microscopic—Swab from lesions, alcohol fix if Pap stain used, otherwise air dry for Giemsa, Tzanck, Wright, direct immunofluorescence (make multiple slides)

Serology—red top tube

Results

Culture—Turnaround is 1–14 days depending on method. Shell vial method results are overnight to 2 days.

Microscopic—Generally less sensitive than culture methods, but if positive the results can be obtained rapidly.

Serology—see below

Clinical Correlation: Asymptomatic shedding of virus during labor has been reported at around 0.20%.

Serology plays a limited role in clinical management as opposed to culture and direct evaluation. A large percentage of adults have positive antibody tests. Differentiation of HSV-1 from HSV-2 is usually not indicated and technically difficult. Recurrent infection may not lead to rising IgG antibody levels.

Asymptomatic or unrecognized viral shedding has been implicated in transmission of genital herpes to more than half of the patients with first episodes of HSV and 50% to 70% of infants with neonatal herpes.

Chronic ulceration persisting greater than one month should lead to consideration of laboratory assessment for AIDS.

HUMAN CHORIONIC GONADOTROPIN (hCG)

Specimen Collection: Serum, urine

Reference Range: Qualitative analysis (negative)
Quantitative analysis (negative = < 5–10 mIU/mL)

Clinical Correlation: Clinically used in

1. Diagnosis of pregnancy
2. Diagnosis of ectopic pregnancy (quantitative levels); patient monitoring following conservative surgery or methotrexate
3. Diagnosis and monitoring in cases of threatened and missed abortions
4. Diagnosis and monitoring of gestational trophoblastic disease
5. Screening for Down syndrome (triple screen with α-fetoprotein and unconjugated estriol)
6. Evaluation of sexual assault
7. Identification of gonadal and extragonadal tumors in the evaluation of sexual precocity

8. Monitoring of patients with ovarian choriocarcinoma, embryonal carcinoma, and other mixed germ cell tumors with trophoblastic differentiation

Serial monitoring of quantitative hCG in early normal pregnancies and abnormal pregnancies:

Levels double approx every 2 days	Normal pregnancy
Levels show a slow rise	Possibly normal
	Possibly ectopic
	Possible loss of one embryo in multiple gestation
Levels show a slow fall	Suspicious for ectopic
Levels show a rapid fall	Nonviable, but less likely as an ectopic

Careful clinical history, physical, and sonographic evaluation in addition to hCG determinations should accompany any woman with suspicion for ectopic pregnancy. Some ectopic pregnancies have shown normal hCG doubling times.

Fossum and colleagues (1) compared the presence of a gestational sac by transvaginal sonography with β-hCG levels. Levels based on the first international reference were 1398 ± 155 mIU/mL. Levels based on the second international reference were 914 ± 106 mIU/mL. Depending on reference standard, hCG measurements in the 1000–1500 mIU/mL range without evidence of a gestational sac in the uterus by transvaginal sonography suggest the possibility of ectopic pregnancy. Patients with symptoms suggesting ectopic pregnancy should have transvaginal sonographic evaluation even if their hCG levels are < 1000 mIU/mL.

Reference

1. Fossum GT, Davajan V, Kletsky OA. Early detection of pregnancy with transvaginal ultrasound. Fertil Steril 1988;49:788–791.

Suggested Reading

Cacciatore B, Stenman UH, Ylostalo P. Diagnosis of ectopic pregnancy by vaginal ultrasonography in combination with a discriminatory serum hCG level of 1000 IU/l (IRP). Br J Obstet Gynaecol 1990;97:904–908.

Heyl PS, Miller W, Canick JA. Maternal serum screening for aneuploid pregnancy by alpha-fetoprotein, hCG, and unconjugated estriol. Obstet Gynecol 1990;76:1025–1031.

Kadar N, Romero R. Further observations on serial human chorionic gonadotropin patterns in ectopic pregnancies and spontaneous abortions. Fertil Steril
1988;50:367–370.

Kadar N, Romero R. Observations on the log human chorionic gonadotropin-time
relationship in early pregnancy and its practical implications. Am J Obstet
Gynecol 1987;157:73–78.

Ory SJ. New options for diagnosis and treatment of ectopic pregnancy. JAMA
1992;267:534–537.

Ory SJ, Villanueva AL, Sand PK, Tamura RK. Conservative treatment of ectopic
pregnancy with methotrexate. Am J Obstet Gynecol 1986;154:1299–1306.

Romero R, Kadar N, Copel JA, Jeanty P, DeCherney AH, Hobbins JC. The value
of serial human chorionic gonadotropin testing as a diagnostic tool in ectopic
pregnancy. Am J Obstet Gynecol 1986;155:392–394.

Seifer DB, Gutmann JN, Doyle MB, Jones EE, Diamond MP, DeCherney AH.
Persistent ectopic pregnancy following laparoscopic linear salpingostomy. Obstet Gynecol 1990;76:1121–1125.

Shepherd RW, Patton PE, Novy MJ, Burry KA. Serial beta-hCG measurements in
the early detection of ectopic pregnancy. Obstet Gynecol 1990;75:417–420.

Suchy SF, Yeager MT. Down syndrome screening in women under 35 with maternal serum hCG. Obstet Gynecol 1990;76:20–24.

van der Lugt B, Drogendijk AC. The disappearance of human chorionic gonadotropin from plasma and urine following induced abortion. Disappearance
of HCG after induced abortion. Acta Obstet Gynecol Scand 1985;64:547–552.

HUMAN IMMUNODEFICIENCY VIRUS (HIV)

Organism: Retrovirus (icosahedral, single-stranded RNA virus), types include HIV-1 and HIV-2.

Transmission: Blood/blood products, sexual exposure, perinatal transmission

Serology: Enzyme-linked immunosorbent assay used initially, false positive
tests occur. Repeat testing and confirmation by Western blot is important.
Antibody negative "window" can extend from a few weeks to 14 months.

Western Blot

Criteria for positivity

Department of Defense—2 or 3 of the following: p24, gp41, and
gp 120/160
Red Cross—one gag, one pol, one env
FDA/Du Pont—p24, p31, and gp41 and/or gp 120/160

HUMAN PAPILLOMAVIRUS (HPV)

Organism: Double-stranded DNA virus, papovavirus family

Specimen Collection: Pap smear, biopsy (cervical, vaginal, vulvar), DNA testing (swab, tissue)

Identification: Cytologic diagnosis on Pap smear is based on koilocytosis. This cytologic change should include not only a distinct space surrounding the nucleus, but also alteration of the nucleus (binucleation-enlargement-irregular nuclear membrane). Hyperkeratosis and parakeratosis are associated but not diagnostic findings.

Histologic diagnosis in the cervix predominantly shows the koilocytes in the intermediate cell layer. Again it is important to have nuclear changes in addition to cytoplasmic space changes to avoid overcalling HPV.

Histologic features of HPV show less koilocytosis on vulvar lesions. Here hyperkeratosis and parakeratosis play more of role in diagnosis. It is important to avoid ascribing an HPV etiology to the small fingerlike squamous papillomata that are typically found on the inner aspect of the labia minora. Hyperkeratosis and parakeratosis are typically absent with a single fibrovascular core present centrally.

Commercially available DNA tests applicable to cytologic and histologic material are available. They are able to screen for three separate groupings of HPV—types (6,11), (16,18), and (31,33, and 35). New testing for additional types is being prepared for clinical use.

Clinical Correlation: The role of molecular testing for HPV in clinical management remains to be defined. Present testing is also positive in patients with latent virus.

Although probes for all types are not commercially available, it is felt that the levels of risk (1) with HPV viral types are represented by the following:

Low risk	6/11, 42,43,44
Intermediate	31,33,35,51,52,58
High-risk "16" group	16
High-risk "18" group	18,45,56

There has been concern with HPV 18. Whereas HPV 16 appears to be equally distributed between dysplastic and cancerous lesions, HPV 18 is found primarily in cancer.

Reference

1. Lorincz AT, Reid R, Jenson AB, Greenberg MD, Lancaster W, Kurman RJ. Human papillomavirus infection of the cervix: relative risk associations of 15 common anogenital types. Obstet Gynecol 1992;79:328–337.

HUMAN PLACENTAL LACTOGEN (HPL)

Clinical Correlation: This placental polypeptide is no longer used for antenatal evaluation, but an immunohistochemical technique that identifies HPL in trophoblastic cells is of value in the diagnosis of placental site trophoblastic tumor.

The identification of trophoblastic cells by HPL determination in passed tissue or uterine curettings is helpful in ruling out ectopic pregnancy when villi cannot be identified. HPL may identify intermediate trophoblastic tissue consistent with intrauterine gestation.

17-HYDROXYPROGESTERONE (17-OHP)

Specimen Collection: Serum, obtain early morning specimen during follicular phase

Reference Range: Normal value is < 2 ng/mL

Clinical Correlation: This test is commonly used in the evaluation of 21-hydroxylase deficiency in women presenting with hyperandrogenism. Elevated values lead to additional testing (see corticotropin stimulation test in Chapter 12 on ambiguous genitalia and Chapter 20 on hyperandrogenism).

IRON STUDIES

Specimen Collection: Serum, fasting morning specimen preferred

Reference Range

Iron	50–132 μg/dL	(9–24 μmol/L)
Iron-binding capacity	265–411 μg/dL	(47–74 μmol/L)

| Iron saturation | 20–55% |
| Transferrin | 200–400 mg/dL   (2.0–3.5 g/L) |

Clinical Correlation: Ferritin determinations have supplanted measurement of iron and iron-binding capacity to a large extent. Iron increases slightly in the first trimester of pregnancy and then falls if the patient is not taking supplements. Iron-binding capacity is increased by about 40% to 50% in pregnancy.

KARYOTYPE

Specimen Collection: Heparin tube for blood sample
    See Chapter 11 (Genetic Analysis of Pregnancy Loss) for information on placental tissue and fetal skin submission to the laboratory.

Clinical Correlation: Karyotype analysis is often performed in the following:

1. For prenatal genetic analysis (chorionic villus sampling, amnio-centesis, fetal blood studies)
2. In the evaluation of pregnancy loss (abortion, stillbirth)
3. In the evaluation of ambiguous genitalia
4. In the evaluation of nonimmune hydrops
5. In the evaluation of younger patients identified with amenorrhea and elevated follicle-stimulating hormone levels.

KETONES, BLOOD AND URINE

Specimen Collection: Serum, urine (random specimen, dipstick evaluation)

Reference Range
    Serum—A positive 1:32 dilution indicates severe ketosis.
    Urine—Semiquantitative results are reported.

Clinical Correlation: Testing is used to evaluate for diabetic ketoacidosis, starvation/hyperemesis in pregnancy.

KLEIHAUER-BETKE (ACID ELUTION FOR FETAL HEMOGLOBIN)

Specimen Collection: EDTA, process immediately, cord blood can provide a positive control

Reference Range: Normal adults have < 0.01% hemoglobin F cells.

Clinical Correlation: Kleihauer-Betke (1) testing is performed in cases where fetal-to-maternal hemorrhage is suspected. It has been reported in trauma, chorangioma, nonimmune hydrops. Quantitative information may guide therapy with D-immune globulin.

A study by Alan Von Stein and colleagues (2) demonstrated positive Kleihauer-Betke tests in 11% of threatened abortions leading the authors to suggest Rho (D) immunoglobulin use in Rho (D)-negative women with this complication.

References

1. Kleihauer E. Determination of fetal hemoglobin: elution technique. In: Schmidt RM, ed. The detection of hemoglobinopathies. Cleveland: CRC Press, 1974.
2. Alan Von Stein G, Munsick RA, Stiver K, Ryder K. Fetomaternal hemorrhage in threatened abortion. Obstet Gynecol 1992;79:383–386.

LACTATE DEHYDROGENASE (LDH) AND ISOENZYMES

Specimen Collection: Serum
Hemolysis interferes with results.

Reference Range: Total LDH—90–180 units/L (levels are slightly elevated in pregnancy)
Isoenzymes by organ and cellular contribution:

Heart muscle—LD-2, LD-1 (LD-1 may predominate over LD-2 or "flipped pattern" may occur with myocardial infarction. LDH peaks later than creatine kinase with myocardial damage.)
Kidney and erythrocytes—LD-1 and LD-2
Platelets, nodes, spleen, lung, and other tissues—LD-2, LD-3, LD-4
Liver and skeletal muscle—LD-4 and LD-5

The electrophoretic *pattern* of the isoenzymes is used for diagnostic purposes.

Clinical Correlation: LDH is an enzyme found in numerous tissues (muscle, liver, red blood cells, kidney, and lung).

LDH and its isoenzymes are used to a limited extent in Ob-Gyn. LDH may be measured as one of the parameters of liver alteration in HELLP (hemolysis, elevated liver enzymes, low platelets) syndrome (levels > 600 units/L).

In gynecologic oncology LDH has proven useful as a tumor marker for dysgerminomas. Increased LDH level may also be indicative of metastatic disease in other malignancies.

LECITHIN/SPHINGOMYELIN RATIO (L/S)

Specimen Collection: Amniotic fluid. Usually requires minimum of 5 mL. Avoid heat and light exposure. Blood and meconium affect results.

Reference Range

<1.5	Immature (respiratory distress in about 70%)
1.5–1.9	Intermediate (respiratory distress in about 40%)
>2.0	Mature (respiratory distress in about 2%)

Clinical Correlation: This is considered the "gold standard" test for fetal lung maturity.

The L/S ratio is performed with either one-dimensional or two-dimensional thin layer chromatography after organic solvent extraction. In these techniques, the density or area of lecithin is compared to sphingomyelin. Lecithin begins to increase rapidly at 34–35 weeks' gestation, while sphingomyelin remains more stable. The two-dimensional technique separates out lecithin, phosphatidylinositol, phosphatidylethanolamine, phosphatidylserine, phosphatidylglycerol, and sphingomyelin. See also Lung Profile test in this section.

The use of sphingomyelin serves as an internal control to help negate the affect of variable amniotic fluid volumes in different patients.

Suggested Reading

Gluck L, Kulovich M, Borer R, Keidel W. The interpretation and significance of the lecithin/sphingomyelin ratio in amniotic fluid. Am J Obstet Gynecol 1974;120:142–155.

Harvey D, Parkinson CE, Campbell S. Risk of respiratory distress syndrome. Lancet 1975;1:42.

LIDOCAINE

Specimen Collection: Serum or plasma

Reference Range: Therapeutic range 1.5–4.0 µg/mL (6.4–17.1 µmol/L)

Clinical Correlation: Toxic levels associated with seizures are usually >
6.0 µg/mL (25.6 µmol/L). This complication of local anesthesia is usually
related to inadvertent intravenous injections.

LIPASE

Specimen Collection: Serum

Reference Range: 4–24 units/dL

Clinical Correlation: Used in conjunction with serum amylase in the diagnosis of pancreatitis.

Listeria monocytogenes

Organism: Gram-positive aerobic motile bacillus

Specimen Collection: Cervical or blood culture, placental or fetal tissue if
death in utero

Identification

Staining methods—Care must be taken not to confuse as diptheroids.
Alert the laboratory to evaluate for this organism.

Serology—complement fixation, fluorescent antibody, enzyme-linked
immunosorbent assay

Clinical Correlation: Maternal infection with *L monocytogenes* is associated with stillbirth, premature labor, neonatal sepsis (early onset), and
neonatal meningitis (late onset). A large outbreak occurred in California in
1985 associated with contaminated cheese (1).

Often the maternal infection is minor. Listeriosis should be part of the
differential in any maternal febrile illness. The neonate is at great risk for
either early onset sepsis or late onset meningitis.

Reference

1. Linnan MJ, Mascola L, Dong Lou X, et al. Epidemic listeriosis associated with
   Mexican-style cheese. N Engl J Med 1988;319:823–828.

LUNG PROFILE

Specimen Collection: Amniotic fluid

Reference Range: Testing reports lecithin/sphingomyelin ratio, percentage of precipitable lecithin, phosphatidylinositol, and phosphatidylglycerol.

Clinical Correlation: The advantage of test is that is also provides information regarding the presence of phosphatidylglycerol, which is not affected by blood or meconium.

Suggested Reading

Kulovich M, Hallman M, Gluck L. The lung profile. Am J Obstet Gynecol 1979;.135:57.

LUPUS ANTICOAGULANT

Specimen Collection: Whole blood (citrate), avoid testing individual recently on heparin or coumadin

Reference Range: Lupus anticoagulant is detected by noting a prolonged activated partial thromboplastin time that is not corrected by the addition of normal plasma. Confirmatory tests include a platelet neutralization method and the Russell viper venom test.

Clinical Correlation: Lupus anticoagulants are IgG or IgM antibodies that prolong phospholipid-dependent coagulation tests. Although it is labeled an anticoagulant, clinically it is related primarily to thrombotic episodes rather than bleeding problems. It is found in 5% to 10% of patients with systemic lupus. Circulating anticoagulants are found in some individuals without autoimmune disease. They have also been found in HIV-positive individuals (1).

Lupus anticoagulant along with anticardiolipin antibodies is associated with pregnancy loss in some women.

Lockwood and colleagues found lupus anticoagulant to be present in 0.2% in a general obstetric population without history of recurrent pregnancy loss (2).

Other circulating anticoagulants may be directed against specific clotting factors (ie, factor VIII antibody in classic hemophilia). Lupus anticoagulant is not directed against a specific factor.

Patients with lupus anticoagulant have a high incidence of false positive syphilis tests.

Circulating anticoagulant has also been identified in the procainamide-induced lupus syndrome (3).

References

1. Taillan B, Roul C, Fuzibet JG, et al. Circulating anticoagulant in patients seropositive for human immunodeficiency virus. Am J Med 1989;87:238.
2. Lockwood CJ, Romero R, Feinberg RF, Clyne LP, Coster B, Hobbins JC. The prevalence and biologic significance of lupus anticoagulant and anticardiolipin antibodies in a general obstetric population. Am J Obstet Gynecol 161:369–373.
3. Bell WR, Boss GR, Wolfson JS. Circulating anticoagulant in the procainamide-induced lupus syndrome. Arch Intern Med 1977;137:1471–1473.

Suggested Reading

Branch DW, Scott JR, Kochenour NK, et al. Obstetric complications associated with the lupus anticoagulant. N Engl J Med 1985;313:1322–1326.
Carp HJ, Frenkel Y, Many A. Fetal demise associated with lupus anticoagulant: clinical features and results of treatment. Gynecol Obstet Invest 1989;28:178–184.
Druzin ML, Lockshin M, Edersheim TG, Hutson JM, Krauss AL, Kogut E. Second-trimester fetal monitoring and preterm delivery in pregnancies with systemic lupus erythematosus and/or circulating anticoagulant. Am J Obstet Gynecol 1987;157:1503–1510.
Hadi HA, Treadwell EL. Lupus anticoagulant and anticardiolipin antibodies in pregnancy: a review. I. Immunochemistry and clinical implications. Obstet Gynecol Surv 1990;45:780–785.
Hadi HA, Treadwell EL. Lupus anticoagulant and anticardiolipin antibodies in pregnancy: a review. II. Diagnosis and management. Obstet Gynecol Surv 1990;45:786–791.
Lubbe WF, Liggins GC. Lupus anticoagulant and pregnancy. Am J Obstet Gynecol 1985;153:322–327.

LUTEINIZING HORMONE (LH)

Specimen Collection: Serum

Reference Range

Women	
Follicular phase	2–15 mIU/mL
Ovulatory peak	13–145 mIU/mL
Luteal phase	2–15 mIU/mL
Postmenopausal	13–145 mIU/mL
Men	7–24 mIU/mL

Clinical Correlation: Clinical correlations for LH testing are found in the following chapters:

1. Amenorrhea (Chapter 18)
2. Ovarian Failure (Chapter 19)
3. Hypothalamic Dysfunction (Chapter 21).
4. Female Fertility (Chapter 22)
5. Male Fertility (Chapter 23)
6. Assisted Reproduction (Chapter 24)
7. Hormonal Assays (Chapter 17)

LH determinations are also performed in the evaluation of precocious puberty.

MAGNESIUM

Specimen Collection: Serum

Reference Range: 1.8–3.0 mg/dL (0.74–1.23 mmol/L)
  Note! 1.0 mEq/L = 1.22 mg/dL
  There is a slight decrease in pregnancy (10%).

Clinical Correlation: The most common use for magnesium levels for the obstetrician is the monitoring of magnesium sulfate therapy for patients manifesting pregnancy-induced hypertension. Laboratory monitoring should always be performed in close conjunction with monitoring of patellar reflexes, respirations, and urinary output. Levels can become significantly elevated in patients with renal compromise. For the patient with normal renal function a magnesium level obtained approximately 4 hours following the loading dose can be used to guide further therapy. The therapeutic level is 4–7 mg/dL. A guide to toxic effects is listed in Chapter 7 on toxicology.

Magnesium levels have been examined in conjunction with the use of magnesium sulfate as a tocolytic for premature labor. Madden and colleagues (1) could not find a good correlation between magnesium levels and tocolytic success.

Reference

1. Madden C, Owen J, Hauth JC. Magnesium tocolysis: serum levels versus success. Am J Obstet Gynecol 1990;162:1177–1180.

MICROVISCOSITY

Specimen Collection: Amniotic fluid
  Blood will interfere with test results.

Reference Range: Maturity correlates with fluorescent polarization levels < 0.321.

Clinical Correlation: This test for fetal maturity using a fluorescent polarization technique is not commonly done, partly due to the expense of the instrumentation. It does have the advantages of being rapid and fairly simple to perform.

Simon and colleagues (1) reported that this test may not be as reliable when used before 34 weeks' gestation.

A variant of methodology is described by Ashwood and Chamberlain (2) whereby fluorescent phosphatidylcholine is used in place of fluorescent diphenylhexatriene.

References

1. Simon NV, Levisky JS, Elser RC, et al. Influence of gestational age on prediction of fetal lung maturity by fluorescence polarization of amniotic fluid. Obstet Gynecol 1985;65:346–351.
2. Ashwood ER, Chamberlain BV. Binding of fluorescent phosphatidylcholine in amniotic fluid. Obstet Gynecol 1988;71:370–374.

Suggested Reading

Barkai G, Mashiach S, Lanzer D, et al. Determination of fetal lung maturity from amniotic fluid microviscosity in high-risk pregnancy. Obstet Gynecol 1982; 59:615–623.
Golde S, Vogt J, Gabbe S, Cabal L. Evaluation of the Felma microviscosimeter in predicting fetal lung maturity. Obstet Gynecol 1979;54:639.

Mobiluncus SPECIES

Organism: Gram-negative bacillus, motile, curved, obligate anaerobe

Clinical Correlation: See Chapter 13 on vulvovaginitis.

MYCOPLASMAS

Organisms: Microorganisms able to grow on cell-free media but lack a cell wall, microaerophilic (clinically relevant organisms include *Mycoplasma hominis, Ureaplasma urealyticum,* and possibly *Mycoplasma genitalium*)

Specimen Collection: Calcium alginate or Dacron swab, specimen should be immediately taken to the laboratory, avoid drying.

Identification: Culture

Clinical Correlation: Both *M hominis* and *U urealyticum* are commonly isolated from asymptomatic females. The organisms are considered as commensals in the lower genital tract. After puberty, colonization with mycoplasmas correlates with sexual activity.

Clinical correlation with disease is presented in the following table. Mycoplasmas have been associated with a number of conditions; proof of causality is difficult to establish with certainty in some of these conditions. Testing for mycoplasmas is not usually performed initially in these conditions.

	M hominis	*U urealyticum*
Upper genital tract infection	association	rarely isolated from tube ? association
Spontaneous abortion	association	association
Chorioamnionitis	association	association
Found in blood culture	+	+
Postpartum endometritis	association	association
Urethral syndrome female	no	association
Urethritis (male)	no	+
Pyelonephritis	+	−
Urinary calculi	−	? association

Rare cases of neonatal meningitis, pneumonia, or skin abscesses have been reported secondary to *M hominis.*

M genitalium has been identified in some men with urethritis, but this organism is difficult to isolate (slow growing).

Carey and colleagues (1) did not find antepartum cultures for *U urealyticum* useful in predicting pregnancy outcome.

There does not appear to be any correlation between mycoplasma infections and the development of prematurity/low birth weight (2).

Both *M hominis* and *U urealyticum* may be tested in couples undergoing infertility evaluation. The clinical benefits for this testing have been debated and some clinicians seek these cultures in second-line evaluations.

References

1. Carey JC, Blackwelder WC, Nugent RP, et al. Antepartum cultures for *Ureaplasma urealyticum* are not useful in predicting pregnancy outcome. The Vaginal Infections and Prematurity Study Group. Am J Obstet Gynecol 1991;164:728–733.
2. Romero R, Mazor M, Oyarzun E, Sirtori M, Wu YK, Hobbins JC. Is genital colonization with *Mycoplasma hominis* or *Ureaplasma urealyticum* associated with prematurity/low birth weight? Obstet Gynecol 1989;73:532–536.

Suggested Reading

Cassell GH, Waites KB, Crouse DT. Perinatal mycoplasmal infections. Clin Perinatol 1991;18:241–262.
Embree J. *Mycoplasma hominis* in maternal and fetal infections. Ann N Y Acad Sci 1988;549:56–64.
Hill AC, Tucker MJ, Whittingham DG, Craft I. Mycoplasmas and in vitro fertilization. Fertil Steril 1987;47:652–655.
Stacey CM, Munday PE, Taylor-Robinson D, et al. A longitudinal study of pelvic inflammatory disease. Br J Obstet Gynaecol 1992;99:994–999.

Neisseria gonorrhoeae

Organism: Gram-negative cocci

Specimen Collection/Transport: Culture sites may include cervix, rectum, urethra, oropharynx, and Bartholin glands. Blood cultures and joint cultures may show isolation of the organism in disseminated gonococcal infection.

The following factors may hinder laboratory diagnosis:

1. Delays in transport
2. Insufficient carbon dioxide
3. Overgrowth of other organisms (ie, proteus or yeast)
4. Vaginal lubricants

Hold culture swab in place 10–15 seconds, collect anorectal specimen from crypts, use selective media such as Thayer-Martin or equivalent. Biplates with different inhibitors in different sections may help increase yield. Use candle jar or CO_2 incubator system, rapid transport to laboratory.

Swab specimen for DNA probe is another analysis method.

Identification: Gram stain—less sensitive in cervical specimens, needs confirmation

Culture, selective media

Coagglutination tests for identification of *N gonorrhoeae* from culture

DNA probe

Clinical Correlation: For additional clinical information see the following chapters:

1. Sexual Assault (Chapter 15)
2. Upper Genital Tract Infections (Chapter 14)
3. Bacterial Infections (Chapter 5)

Follow-up cultures are usually performed 4–7 days after therapy to assess for resistant organisms and treatment failure.

NITRAZINE TESTING

Specimen Collection: Vaginal pool fluid, avoid the cervix

Clinical Correlation: Amniotic fluid is alkaline and will turn the paper blue.

False positive results may result from alkalinity associated with trichomonas, blood, or cervical mucus.

False negative results may occur if the amount of amniotic fluid is scant and/or a prolonged time period has elapsed since rupture.

Suggested Reading

Gorodeski IG, Haimovitz L, Bahari CM. Reevaluation of the pH, ferning, and nile blue sulphate staining methods in pregnant women with premature rupture of the fetal membranes. J Perinat Med 1982;10:286.

Smith R. A technique for the detection of rupture of the membranes. A review and preliminary report. Obstet Gynecol 1976;48:172–176.

OSMOLALITY, SERUM AND URINE

Specimen Collection: Serum
Random or timed urine specimen

Reference Range

Serum	280–290 mOsm/kg (280–290 mmol/kg)
Urine	250–900 mOsm/kg (250–900 mmol/kg)

Clinical Correlation: Clinical use of serum osmolality is in the evaluation of electrolyte and fluid balance, antidiuretic hormone function, seizures, and coma.

Clinical use of urine osmolality is in the evaluation of kidney concentrating ability, antidiuretic hormone function, and diabetes insipidus.

OVA AND PARASITES

Organisms: Intestinal parasitic organisms more commonly seen in the United States include *Ascaris lumbricoides, Necator americanus, Diphyllobothrium latum, Taenia saginata, Entamoeba histolytica,* and *Giardia lamblia.*

Specimen Collection: Warm saline or Fleet enema specimens acceptable, but recent barium, mineral oil, and certain laxatives may obscure results. Avoid contamination of specimen with urine or toilet water. Stools that cannot reach the laboratory within one hour should be refrigerated and preserved in formalin. Multiple specimens are usually performed. Be very careful with all specimens due to infectivity of some of the organisms.

Identification: Wet and stained preparations performed
Immunofluorescence and enzyme-linked immunosorbent assay may help in identification.

Clinical Correlation: See also Chapter 6 on fungal and parasitic infections and *Enterobius vermicularis* in this section.

OVARIAN ANTIBODIES

Clinical Correlation: Testing availability limited to specialty laboratories and university centers. See Chapter 19 on ovarian failure.

PAP SMEAR

Specimen Collection: Ectocervical and endocervical sample, rapid fixation, avoid lubricants, blood, and excess discharge.

Removing excess mucus from the canal may help in better endocervical sampling.

Reference Range: Bethesda system is now being used by most laboratories. Older classifications were modifications of Papanicolaou's numbered system.

Clinical Correlation

Adequacy

Some slide preparations are clearly unsatisfactory due to obscuring factors (blood, inflammation, lubricant, cytolysis) and quantity of material (too thick a spread, scanty specimen). Presently the differential between "satisfactory" and "satisfactory but limited . . ." depends on individual laboratories and screeners. A guide will be forthcoming from the Bethesda group to try to obtain more uniformity. Whether the clinician elects to repeat a satisfactory but limited smear may depend on the individual patient circumstance.

Infections

Although the principal purpose of the Pap smear is to screen for premalignant and malignant cells, identification of infectious organisms is additionally helpful for the clinician. Yeast, trichomonads, herpes infection, *Actinomyces* species, and the general bacterial pattern can be observed on the cytology preparation. If the clinician receives a report describing trichomonads in a patient in whom there is not good clinical confirmatory evidence, it is probably best to perform a wet smear preparation. Sometimes cellular fragments may be overinterpreted. There is not enough information presently to decide if the cytology report will greatly benefit the pregnant patient in regard to bacterial pattern. Culture studies have looked at non-Lactobacillus patterns and pregnancy complications.

Epithelial abnormalities

Most clinicians will recommend colposcopy for reports identifying atypical squamous cells of undetermined significance if the cytopathologist favors neoplastic change. Colposcopy is also performed for low-grade, high-grade, and malignant "squamous" smears.

Atypical glandular cells of undetermined significance may prove to be a reactive process on histologic follow-up, but the possibility of endocervical adenocarcinoma (in situ and invasive), a squamous lesion replacing the endocervical glands, or a glandular lesion from higher in the genital tract should all be considered. Pap smear identification of endometrial cells out of phase or in a postmenopausal patient warrants a clinical review of the patient's menstrual cycle, medications, etc and consideration of endometrial biopsy.

Hormonal evaluation

Hormonal patterns on Pap smears provide the clinician with estrogen status. In rare cases a smear may identify abnormal estrogen production in a postmenopausal patient (not taking hormone replacement).

PARATHYROID HORMONE (PTH)

Specimen Collection: Serum

Reference Range: Laboratory levels will vary according to technique used. It is important to know which PTH component is being measured (intact, C-terminal, N-terminal).

Clinical Correlation: This test is used for evaluation of parathyroid disorders and hypercalcemia.

Evaluation of PTH is performed with concurrent testing of calcium, phosphorus, and creatinine. The general relationship with calcium is the following:

High PTH, low calcium—secondary hyperparathyroidism
Low PTH, low calcium—hypoparathyroidism
High PTH, high calcium—primary hyperparathyroidism
Low PTH, high calcium—nonparathyroid mediated hypercalcemia
(ie, neoplasm)

See Chapter 19 on ovarian failure and the discussion of parathyroid hypofunction in association with ovarian failure.

PARVOVIRUS (B19)

Organism: Single-stranded DNA virus

Specimen Collection: Serum for serologic testing
Amniotic fluid, fetal blood (cordocentesis)

Identification

Serology—IgM-specific antibody using immunoassay (IgG is found in 30% to 50% of healthy adults).

DNA testing—Hybridization methods (including polymerase chain reaction) have been used for diagnosis.

Clinical Correlation: Associated with erythema infectiosum ("fifth disease"), occasional severe anemias, arthritis, hydrops fetalis, and fetal death
Cordocentesis laboratory results can help to guide therapy (1,2).

Anemia is a manifestation of the viral replication within developing red cells.

References

1. Sahakian V, Weiner CP, Naides SJ, Williamson RA, Scharosch LL. Intrauterine transfusion treatment of nonimmune hydrops fetalis secondary to human parvovirus B19 infection. Am J Obstet Gynecol 1991;164:1090–1091.
2. Peters MT, Nicolaides KH. Cordocentesis for the diagnosis and treatment of human fetal parvovirus infection. Obstet Gynecol 1990;75:501–504.

PATERNITY TESTING

Specimen Collection: Serum; careful attention must be paid to establish that the results are admissible in court (witnesses, photographs, proper labeling and signatures).

Laboratory Procedures: Tests used will depend on local laws concerning acceptable evidence; they may include evaluation of red cell antigens (ABO, MNS, Rh, Kell, Duffy, etc) and HLA typing.

More recently, the additional use of DNA technology offers greater accuracy in testing (restriction fragment length polymorphisms, probes that detect tandem repeats, and multilocus probes; 1–3).

Reference Range: Reports are usually given as paternity index, which is a numerical ratio of the frequency that the alleged father could produce sperm with the obligatory genes compared to a random man of the same racial group. Conversion to a probability of paternity expressed as a percentage is then derived.

Clinical Correlation: Paternity analysis can also be performed in early pregnancy using chorionic villus sampling (4).

References

1. Helminen P, Ehnholm C, Lokki ML, Jeffreys A, Peltonen L. Application of DNA "fingerprints" to paternity determinations. Lancet 1988;1:574–576.

2. Jeffreys AJ, Turner M, Debenham P. The efficiency of multilocus DNA fingerprint probes for individualization and establishment of family relationships, determined from extensive casework. Am J Hum Genet 1991;48:824–840.
3. Smouse PE, Chakraborty R. The use of restriction fragment length polymorphisms in paternity analysis. Am J Hum Genet 1986;38:918–939.
4. Kovacs BW, Shahbahrami B, Medearis AL, Comings DE. Prenatal determinations of paternity by molecular genetic "fingerprinting." Obstet Gynecol 1990;75:474–479.

Suggested Reading

Kolins MD, Walker RH. Laboratory determination of parentage. Obstet Gynecol Surv 1988;43:590–595.

PERITONEAL FLUID, CYTOLOGIC EXAMINATION

Specimen Collection: Washings at the time of laparoscopy, laparotomy

Clinical Correlation: Primarily used in Ob-Gyn for detection of malignant cells.

Cytologic evaluation is sometimes difficult due to the presence of atypical reactive mesothelial cells.

Cytologic evidence of malignant cells is important in management considerations for ovarian and endometrial malignancies. Only rare cases of cervical carcinoma have peritoneal manifestations.

Suggested Reading

McLellan R, Dillon MB, Currie JL, Rosenshein NB. Peritoneal cytology in endometrial cancer: a review. Obstet Gynecol Surv 1989;44:711–719.

pH, FETAL SCALP

Specimen Collection: Blood sample obtained through vaginal endoscope. Cervix needs to be significantly dilated. Scalpel is cleaned with a swab and coated with silicone to allow beading of blood. Incision is made to 2 mm depth. Care is taken to avoid clotting in heparinized capillary tube.

Reference Range: pH normally > 7.25

Clinical Correlation: Fetal scalp pH measurements are used by clinicians in *select* situations to assess the fetal status. Close observation has been given to levels in the 7.20–7.25 range with follow-up levels obtained within 30 minutes. Levels < 7.20 may be indicative of fetal distress. pH levels are also influenced by maternal acid-base status.

Suggested Reading

Bowen LW, Kochenour NK, Rehm NE, Woolley FR. Maternal-fetal pH difference and fetal scalp pH as predictors of neonatal outcome. Obstet Gynecol 1986;67:487.

Clark SL, Paul RH. Intrapartum fetal surveillance. The role of fetal scalp sampling. Am J Obstet Gynecol 1985;153:717.

pH, VAGINAL FLUID

Specimen Collection: Obtain sample of discharge from lateral vaginal wall with a swab. Recent intercourse and douching can alter the results. Some strips are available that are less light sensitive and have a long shelf life (colorpHast®).

Reference Range: Normally < 4.5

Clinical Correlation:
pH correlates

< 4.5	Normal, yeast
4.5–6.0	Bacterial vaginosis
> 6.0	Contamination with cervical mucus, *Trichomonas*

PHEOCHROMOCYTOMA TESTING

Tests and Reference Ranges: 24-hour urine determination

Metanephrines, total	0.3–0.9 mg/24 h	(1.5–4.6 µmol/d)
Vanillylmandelic acid	< 7.0 mg/24 h	(<35 µmol/d)
Urinary catecholamines	<100 µg/24 h	(<590 nmol/d)

Other tests include plasma catecholamines and 3,4-dihydroxyphenyglycol, but urine testing is performed initially to screen.

Clinical Correlation: These tests are used for diagnosis of pheochromocytoma. This rare tumor, which typically causes hypertension, can arise in the adrenal medulla or numerous extradrenal sites. Fatal hypertensive crises can occur. Some pheochromocytomas are malignant and can metastasize. The discussion of this tumor is pertinent to Ob-Gyn because it can simulate symptoms of pregnancy-induced hypertension. Maternal deaths from this tumor have been primarily women who were undiagnosed before delivery. Clues to proceeding with laboratory investigation include:

1. Paroxysmal hypertension, headaches, palpitations, and sweating
2. Hypertension without proteinuria or edema
3. Hypertension refractory to therapy
4. Family history of pheochromocytoma or multiple endocrine neoplasia

PHOSPHATIDYLGLYCEROL (PG)

Specimen Collection: Amniotic fluid (the quantity of fluid needed for the agglutination assay is less than the chromatography method, 1.0 mL compared to 5.0 mL)

Reference Range: Slide agglutination method can detect 2 μg/mL concentration of PG. The advantage of this test is its ability to be used with amniotic fluid obtained from vaginal specimens and less interference with blood and meconium.

Clinical Correlation: Appearing initially at around 35 weeks' gestation and rapidly increasing in succeeding weeks

The slide agglutination method (Amniostat-FLM®) has shown good concordance with the thin-layer chromatography method, especially when the chromatography method demonstrates > 3% phosphatidylglycerol.

Suggested Reading

Halvorsen PR, Gross TL. Laboratory and clinical evaluation of a rapid slide agglutination test for phosphatidylglycerol. Am J Obstet Gynecol 1985;151:1061–1066.

PHOSPHORUS

Specimen Collection: Serum

Reference Range: 2.5–5.0 mg/dL (0.8–1.60 mmol/L); no significant change in pregnancy

Clinical Correlation: For use in conjunction with calcium determination to evaluate for parathyroid disorders.

Phthirus pubis

Organism: Louse

Specimen Collection: Usually present in pubic area, but rarely may be found in axilla, scalp, eyelashes

Identification: Shorter and crablike in comparison to body and head lice After a blood meal the lice are rust colored and more easily identified. Microscopy can distinguish empty nits from those containing developing nymph.

Clinical Correlation: Primarily a sexually transmitted organism that may lead to symptoms of pruritus or rust colored staining of underclothes.

Suggested Reading

Long JG. Infestations. In: Morse SA, Moreland AA, Thompson SE, eds. Atlas of sexually transmitted diseases. Philadelphia: JB Lippincott, 1990.

PLACENTAL CULTURE

Specimen Collection: For the vaginally delivered placenta in cases of suspected chorioamnionitis, sterilize the fetal surface, incise the surface membrane, and obtain swab specimen just beneath the surface. This procedure is intended to decrease the amount of vaginal contaminants.

PLATELET COUNT

Specimen Collection: EDTA

Reference Range:
$150–400 \times 10^3/\mu L$ ($150–400 \times 10^9/L$)
The platelet count decreases slightly in pregnancy.

Clinical Correlation: Platelet count determinations are performed in the following:

1. Preeclampsia
2. Consumptive coagulopathy (septicemia, abruptio)
3. Bleeding complications of pregnancy/massive blood transfusion
4. Immune thrombocytopenic purpura (idiopathic)

5. Patients on heparin therapy
6. Patients receiving chemotherapy
7. Monitoring patients with lupus during pregnancy

Different laboratory parameters have been studied to assess the risk of neonatal thrombocytopenia in the infants of mothers with immunologic thrombocytopenic purpura. Maternal counts do not correlate well with fetal platelet counts. Circulating platelet antibody (1), platelet-associated antibody (2), and more recently indirect platelet antiglobulin (3) have been assessed as a maternal predictor of fetal risk. Direct evaluation of fetal platelets has been obtained with scalp sampling and umbilical cord blood sampling.

References

1. Cines DB, Dusak B, Tomaski A, Mennuti M, Schreier AD. Immune thrombocytopenic purpura and pregnancy. N Engl J Med 1982;306:826–831.
2. Kelton JG, Inwood MJ, Barr RM, et al. The prenatal prediction of thrombocytopenia in infants of mothers with clinically diagnosed immune thrombocytopenia. Am J Obstet Gynecol 1982;144:449–454.
3. Samuels P, Bussel JB, Braitman LE, et al. Estimation of the risk of thrombocytopenia in the offspring of pregnant women with presumed immune thrombocytopenic purpura. N Engl J Med 1990;323:229–235.

PLATELETS FOR TRANSFUSION

Specimen Collection: Separated from donated whole blood or obtained from apheresis

Random-donor platelets (from a unit of whole blood)—$6\text{--}8 \times 10^9$ platelets/bag containing 50–70 mL plasma

Apheresis unit—$3\text{--}6 \times 10^{11}$ platelets/bag containing 200–400 mL plasma

Storage: 20°–24°C

Important to keep pH above 6.0.

Shelf life is 3–5 days.

Freezing is possible with storage for up to 3 years. There is a loss of platelets with the freeze-thaw process.

Clinical Correlation: Generally given to markedly thrombocytopenic patients with levels < 20,000/μL. A level of 50,000/μL is considered for transfusion if surgery is contemplated.

One unit of platelets will raise the platelet count by 5–10,000/µL; therefore, it takes approximately 4–6 units to have clinical significance.

Adverse reactions include:

1. Bacterial contamination
2. Transmission of hepatitis, HIV, malaria
3. Fluid overload if multiple units given
4. Febrile reactions secondary to proteins or leukocytes
5. Graft-versus-host disease in immunocompromised patients if lymphocytes present
6. Rh sensitization; therefore, platelet transfusions should be ABO and Rh specific

Pneumocystis carinii

Organism: Unclassified but thought to be protozoal

Specimen Collection: Sputum, pulmonary washings, lung tissue

Identification: Silver, Giemsa, toluidine blue staining methods for microscopic diagnosis

Clinical Correlation: See Chapter 6 on fungal and parasitic infections.

POLYMERASE CHAIN REACTION

Methodology: A method allowing large amounts of DNA sequences to be synthesized over a short period of time

Clinical Correlation: Numerous clinical applications in the evaluation of genetically related disease and infections

PROGESTERONE

Specimen Collection: Serum

Reference Range

Preovulatory	<1 ng/mL	(3.2 nmol/L)
Midluteal	10–20 ng/mL	(31.8–63.6 nmol/L)

Clinical Correlation: Progesterone determinations have been performed to evaluate ectopic and aborting pregnancies. Levels > 25 ng/mL have generally been associated with normally developing intrauterine pregnancies. Levels $\leq$ 5–15 ng/mL have been associated with ectopic and nonviable pregnancies. There has been some debate on the clinical value of the test (1).

Progesterone levels have been studied as predictors of in vitro fertilization success (2).

Midluteal progesterone determinations > 5 ng/mL are consistent with ovulation.

References

1. Peterson CM, Kreger D, Delgado P, Hung TT. Laboratory and clinical comparison of a rapid versus a classic progesterone radioimmunoassay for use in determining abnormal and ectopic pregnancies. Am J Obstet Gynecol 1992; 166:562–566.
2. Silverberg KM, Burns WN, Olive DL, Riehl RM, Schenken RS. Serum progesterone levels predict success of in vitro fertilization/embryo transfer in patients stimulated with leuprolide acetate and human menopausal gonadotropins. J Clin Endocrinol Metab 1991;73:797–803.

PROLACTIN

Specimen Collection: Serum, mid morning collection

Reference Range: < 20 ng/mL (20 µg/L)

Clinical Correlation: For clinical correlations see the following chapters:

1. Amenorrhea (Chapter 18)
2. Hyperandrogenism (Chapter 20)
3. Hypothalamic Dysfunction (Chapter 21)

PROTEIN, URINE

Specimen Collection: Random urine for qualitative dipstick evaluation
24-hour urine collection for quantitative level
Interfering factors may include:

1. Excessive physical activity
2. Diets containing large amounts of protein

3. Contaminated specimens from vaginal discharge or blood
4. Alkaline and dilute urine specimens

Reference Range

Dipstick—negative (trace results at 100–200 mg/L)
24-hour urine—50–80 mg/24 hours

Clinical Correlation: Urinary evaluation of protein is one of the principle tests in the diagnosis of renal disease. Proteinuria usually implicates glomerular damage and increased filtration. Urinary protein consists of albumin and globulins. Albumin is filtered more readily and can appear in significant amounts in certain types of renal disease.

Urinary protein determinations (dipstick) augment the evaluation of weight gain, edema, and blood pressure for detection of preeclampsia. Proteinuria is identified if 300 mg or more of protein is found in a 24-hour collection.

Urinary protein determinations are also performed in pregnant patients with chronic renal disease, insulin-dependent diabetes, and systemic lupus erythematosus.

PROTHROMBIN TIME (PT)

Specimen Collection: Whole blood, sodium citrate, completely fill, invert to mix

Reference Range: 10.6–12.9 seconds (no significant change in pregnancy)

Clinical Correlation: This test is a measure of the extrinsic portion of the coagulation cascade.

The PT is prolonged if extrinsic factor levels are < 50% of normal or if the fibrinogen is < 100 mg/dL.

Prolongation of PT occurs most often clinically in liver disease, disseminated intravascular coagulation, vitamin K deficiency, and in the clinical use of oral anticoagulants (warfarin).

PT is used to monitor oral anticoagulant therapy. Interlaboratory comparison of PT results is difficult due to the use of different reagents. Standardization has been attempted by use of the International Normalized Ratio (INR).

RETICULOCYTE COUNT

Specimen Collection: EDTA

Reference Range: 0.5% to 1.5% (some use a slightly higher percentage for menstruating women). Reticulocyte count is elevated slightly in pregnancy.

Clinical Correlation: The reticulocyte is the red blood cell that has recently lost its nucleus but retains a reticulin-like network of RNA. With stimulation of red cell production reticulocytes are prematurely released into the blood stream. An elevated reticulocyte count thus gives an indication of increased production when the clinician is evaluating a normocytic anemia.

A low reticulocyte count does not rule out blood loss or hemolysis. A markedly low count usually corresponds to marrow suppression.

Weiner and associates established patterns for predicting fetal anemia and establishing the timing of repeat cordocentesis using reticulocyte counts and direct Coombs' tests (1).

Reticulocyte counts are used to monitor lupus patients during pregnancy. Reticulocytosis may also be present when fragmentation hemolysis is present in hypertensive disease in pregnancy.

Reference

1. Weiner CP, Williamson RA, Wenstrom KD, Sipes SL, Grant SS, Widness JA. Management of fetal hemolytic disease by cordocentesis. I. Prediction of fetal anemia. Am J Obstet Gynecol 1991;165:546–553.

ROSETTE TEST, ERYTHROCYTE

Specimen Collection: EDTA

Reference Range: No rosetting is seen if Rho (D) fetal cells are absent.

Clinical Correlation: See Chapter 8 on erythroblastosis fetalis.

RUBELLA

Organism: Single-stranded RNA virus

Transmission/Incubation: Nasopharyngeal secretions transmission to children and adults; intrauterine transmission to fetus / incubation is 7–10 days.

Specimen Collection

Culture—throat swab, urine, placenta, blood, stool
Serology—red top tube

Results

Culture—Turnaround is 10–14 days.
Serology—Hemagglutination inhibition titer $\geq$ 1:8 is considered immune. Acute infection is diagnosed by rising titers.

Clinical Correlation: Culture methods are used to diagnose congenital rubella in the infant and in monitoring the duration of virus excretion.

Serology is used to establish maternal immune status and aid in diagnosing acute infection.

Sarcoptes scabiei

Organism: Mite

Specimen Collection: The specimen may be identified after scraping the suspect burrow with a scalpel.

Identification: Can be made by finding the adult, larva, or eggs microscopically. Central protruding jaws flanked by four legs are clues to the diagnosis. The back pairs of legs may be more difficult to distinguish. Burrows can be detected through ink or Wood's light techniques.

Clinical Correlation: The mite, *S scabiei,* is the causative agent for a pruritic dermatosis. Skin contact that may or may not be associated with intercourse will spread the mite. The female burrows into the stratum corneum to lay eggs. The body distribution of the mites includes axilla, elbow, wrist, finger webs, belt line, genital, anal, knee, and foot regions. Secondary bacterial infections can occur in the infected sites.

Suggested Reading

Long JG. Infestations. In: Morse SA, Moreland AA, Thompson SE, eds. Atlas of sexually transmitted diseases. Philadelphia: JB Lippincott, 1990.

SEMEN ANALYSIS

See Chapter 23 on male fertility.

SHAKE TEST

Specimen Collection: Amniotic fluid
   The test may be altered by blood, meconium, and amniotic fluid volume.

Reference Range: Maturity is correlated with finding a complete stable ring of bubbles 15 minutes after shaking a 1:2 amniotic fluid dilution for 15 seconds.

Clinical Correlation: This fetal lung maturity test evaluates the ability of surfactant to form a stable foam in the presence of ethanol. Careful technique is essential for this test, with correct ethanol concentration and clean glassware critical for proper evaluation.
   See also Foam Stability Index (Lumadex) in this section.

Suggested Reading

Clements JA, Platzker A, Tierney D, et al. Assessment of the risk of the respiratory-distress syndrome by a rapid test for surfactant in amniotic fluid. N Engl J Med 1972;286:1081.

SPECIFIC GRAVITY

Specimen Collection: Random urine

Clinical Correlation: Test used to evaluate renal concentrating function
   Elevated (> 1.020) in dehydration, vomiting, diarrhea, diabetes (glucosuria), syndrome of inappropriate antidiuretic hormone, and with proteinuria
   Decreased (< 1.009) with glomerulonephritis, pyelonephritis, excess fluids, diuresis
   Fixed (1.010) with severe renal damage

SPERM ANTIBODY TESTING

Specimen Collection: Specimens may include serum from both the male and female, semen, and cervical mucus.

Methodology: A number of methods have been reported, including sperm agglutination, sperm immobilization, immunobead testing, mixed antiglobulin reaction assay, microcytotoxicity, dot-immunoblot, enzyme-linked immunosorbent assays, and flow cytometry.

Clinical Correlation: See Chapter 23 on male fertility.

Though some feel that this testing is not helpful, indications used by others include:

1. Poor postcoital tests (immobilized sperm, no progressive motility, or no sperm with normal semen analysis)
2. Poor sperm penetration assay

Sperm antibodies develop in men who have undergone vasectomy, have had a testicular biopsy and have a history of cryptorchid testes.

The immunobead test has largely supplanted some of the older agglutinating and immobilizing tests. Different classes of antibodies on different regions of motile sperm can be evaluated with this test.

Suggested Reading

Alexander NJ, Alexander DJ. Vasectomy: consequences of autoimmunity to sperm antigens. Fertil Steril 1979;32:253.

Bandoh R, Yamano S, Kamada M, Daitoh T, Aono T. Effect of sperm-immobilizing antibodies on the acrosome reaction of human spermatozoa. Fertil Steril 1992;57:387–392.

Bronson R, Cooper G, Hjort T, et al. Antisperm antibodies detected by agglutination, immobilization, microcytotoxicity, and immunobead-binding assays. J Reprod Immunol 1985;8:279–299.

Clark GN, Elliott PJ, Smaila C. Detection of sperm antibodies in semen using the immunobead test: a survey of 813 consecutive patients. Am J Reprod Immunol 1985;7:118–123.

Franklin RR, Dukes CD. Antispermatozoal antibody and unexplained infertility. Am J Obstet Gynecol 1964;89:6.

Friberg J. Relation between sperm-agglutinating antibodies in serum and seminal fluid. Acta Obstet Gynecol Scand (Suppl) 1974;36:73.

Haas GG Jr. Antibody-mediated causes of male infertility. Urol Clin North Am 1987;14:539–550.

Hellstrom WJ, Samuels SJ, Waits AB, Overstreet JW. A comparison of the usefulness of SpermMar and immunobead tests for the detection of antisperm antibodies. Fertil Steril 1989;52:1027–1031.

Isojima S, Li TS, Ashitaka Y. Immunologic analysis of sperm-immobilizing factor found in sera of women with unexplained sterility. Am J Obstet Gynecol 1968;101:677.

Mandelbaum SL, Diamond MP, DeCherney AH. The impact of antisperm antibodies on human infertility. J Urol 1987;138:1–8.

Menge AC, Beitner O. Interrelationships among semen characteristics, antisperm antibodies, and cervical mucus penetration assays in infertile human couples. Fertil Steril 1989;51:486–492.

Nikolaeva MA, Kulakov VI, Ter-Avanesov GV, Terekhina LN, Pshenichnikova TJ, Sukhikh GT. Detection of antisperm antibodies on the surface of living spermatozoa using flow cytometry: preliminary study. Fertil Steril 1993;59:639–644.

Rajah SV, Parslow JM, Howell RJ, Hendry WF. Comparison of mixed antiglobulin reaction and direct immunobead test for detection of sperm-bound antibodies in subfertile males. Fertil Steril 1992;57:1300–1303.

Rousseaux-Prevost R, De Almeida M, Hublau P, et al. Antibodies to sperm basic nuclear proteins detected in infertile patients by dot-immunoblotting assay and by enzyme-linked immunosorbent assay. Am J Reprod Immunol 1989;20:17–20.

Shulman S, Hu C. A study of the detection of sperm antibody in cervical mucus with a modified immunobead method. Fertil Steril 1992;58:387–391.

Stern JE, Dixon PM, Manganiello PD, Brinck-Johnsen T. Antisperm antibodies in women: variability in antibody levels in serum, mucus, and peritoneal fluid. Fertil Steril 1992;58:950–958.

SPERM PENETRATION ASSAY

Specimen Collection: Semen

Reference Range: Many of the studies list abnormal results as $< 10\%$ to 15% of eggs penetrated.

Clinical Correlation: See Chapter 23 on male fertility.

Suggested Reading

Bronson RA, Rogers BJ. Pitfalls of the zona-free hamster egg penetration test: protein source as a major variable. Fertil Steril 1988;50:851–854.

Falk RM, Silverberg KM, Fetterolf PM, Kirchner FK, Rogers BJ. Establishment of TEST-yolk buffer enhanced sperm penetration assay limits for fertile males. Fertil Steril 1990;54:121–126.

Mao C, Grimes DA. The sperm penetration assay: can it discriminate between fertile and infertile men? Am J Obstet Gynecol 1988;159:279–286.

Margalioth EJ, Bronson RA, Cooper GW, Rosenfeld DL. Luteal phase sera and progesterone enhance sperm penetration in the hamster egg assay. Fertil Steril 1988;50:117–122.

Margalioth EJ, Feinmesser M, Navot D, Mordel N, Bronson RA. The long-term predictive value of the zona-free hamster ova sperm penetration assay. Fertil Steril 1989;52:490–494.

Smith RG, Johnson A, Lamb D, Lipshultz LI. Functional tests of spermatozoa. Sperm penetration assay. Urol Clin North Am 1987;14:451–458.

Staphylococcus aureus

Organism: Gram-positive coccus

Specimen collection: Wound culture, blood culture

Identification: Gram stain, culture

Clinical Correlation: *S aureus* infections and sequelae in Ob-Gyn may include:

Wound infections and abscess
Toxic shock syndrome
Mastitis and breast abscess
Osteitis pubis
Postabortal infection
Septicemia

S aureus toxins—Toxic shock syndrome toxin-1 (TSST-1) and staphylococcal enterotoxin B (SEB) are associated with a devastating multisystem illness named toxic shock syndrome. Prominent clinical manifestations include hypotension, high fever, erythematous rash, vomiting, diarrhea, mucous membrane hyperemia, and altered consciousness. Other laboratory abnormalities may include decreased white cell counts, elevated creatine phosphokinase, blood urea nitrogen, creatinine and alanine aminotransferase, and thrombocytopenia.

Suggested Reading

Bowen LW, Sand PK, Ostergard DR. Toxic shock syndrome following carbon dioxide laser treatment of genital tract *Condyloma acuminatum*. Am J Obstet Gynecol 1986;154:145–146.

Centers for Disease Control: Toxic shock syndrome, United States, 1970–1982. MMWR 1982;31:201.

Demey HE, Hautekeete ML, Buytaert P, Bossaert LL. Mastitis and toxic shock syndrome. Acta Obstet Gynecol Scand 1989;68:87–88.

Friedell S, Mercer LJ. Nonmenstrual toxic shock syndrome. Obstet Gynecol Surv 1986;41:336–341.

Todd JK. Toxic shock syndrome. Clin Microbiol Rev 1989;1:432.

Wiesenthal AM, Ressman M, Caston SA, Todd JK. Toxic shock syndrome. I. Clinical exclusion of other syndromes by strict and screening definitions. Am J Epidemiol 1985;122:847–856.

Staphylococcus saprophyticus

Organism: Gram-positive coccus

Specimen Collection: Urine culture

Identification: Culture

Clinical Correlation: *S saprophyticus* is found in approximately 10% to 15% of urinary tract infections.

Streptococcus agalactiae (GROUP B STREPTOCOCCUS, GBS)

Organism: Gram-positive cocci

Specimen Collection: Cervical culture, blood culture

Identification: Gram stain, culture
   Rapid detection methods include use of a starch broth culture to detect a pigment change, a coagglutination method, latex agglutination, enzyme-linked immunosorbent assay, electroimmunoassay.

Clinical Correlation: Clinically associated with chorioamnionitis, maternal and neonatal sepsis (early and late onset infections), and postpartum endomyometritis. There have been case reports of mastitis and of fetal death in utero (following funipuncture) related to GBS.
   Asymptomatic carriage is common.
   Routine prenatal screening for the organism is not recommended.
   Culture for GBS is performed in cases of preterm labor and premature rupture of membranes. The clinical benefits of culture are limited by timeliness of results. Culture results may also be altered by recent rupture of membranes.
   Gram staining for GBS lacks sensitivity and specificity.
   Rapid immunoassay methods to detect GBS are hampered by some false positive as well as false negative results. The test performance improves when moderate to large amounts of organisms are present. Negative predictive values are better than positive predictive values for many of the

tests. Newer test methodologies involving DNA probes may allow for identification of the patient with lighter colonization with GBS.

Suggested Reading

Armer T, Clark P, Duff P, Saravanos K. Rapid intrapartum detection of group B streptococcal colonization with an enzyme immunoassay. Am J Obstet Gynecol 1993;168:39–43.

Carey JC, Klebanoff MA, Regan JA. Evaluation of the Gram stain as a screening tool for maternal carriage of group B beta-hemolytic streptococci. The Vaginal Infections and Prematurity Study Group. Obstet Gynecol 1990;76:693–697.

Gentry YM, Hillier SL, Eschenbach DA. Evaluation of a rapid enzyme immuno-assay test for detection of group B streptococcus. Obstet Gynecol 1991;78:397–401.

Greenspoon JS, Fishman A, Wilcox JG, Greenspoon RL, Lewis W. Comparison of culture for group B streptococcus versus enzyme immunoassay and latex agglu-tination rapid tests: results in 250 patients during labor. Obstet Gynecol 1991;77:97–100.

Greenspoon JS, Wilcox JG, Kirschbaum TH. Group B streptococcus: the effec-tiveness of screening and chemoprophylaxis. Obstet Gynecol Surv 1991;46:499–508.

Hagay ZJ, Miskin A, Goldchmit R, Federman A, Matzkel A, Mogilner BM. Eval-uation of two rapid tests for detection of maternal endocervical group B strepto-coccus: enzyme-linked immunosorbent assay and Gram stain. Obstet Gynecol 1993;82:84–87.

Henderson CE, Egre H, Turk R, Aning V, Szilagyi G, Divon MY. Amniorrhexis lowers the incidence of positive cultures for group B streptococci. Am J Obstet Gynecol 1993;168:624–625.

McColgin SW, Hess LW, Martin RW, Martin JN Jr, Morrison JC. Group B strepto-coccal sepsis and death in utero following funipuncture. Obstet Gynecol 1989;74:464–465.

Skoll MA, Mercer BM, Baselski V, Gray JP, Ryan G, Sibai BM. Evaluation of two rapid group B streptococcal antigen tests in labor and delivery patients. Obstet Gynecol 1991;77:322–326.

Towers CV, Garite TJ, Friedman WW, Pircon RA, Nageotte MP. Comparison of a rapid enzyme-linked immunosorbent assay test and the Gram stain for detec-tion of group B streptococcus in high-risk antepartum patients. Am J Obstet Gynecol 1990;163:965–967.

Yancey MK, Clark P, Armer T, Duff P. Use of a DNA probe for the rapid detection of group B streptococci in obstetric patients. Obstet Gynecol 1993;81:635–640.

Streptococcus pyogenes (GROUP A STREPTOCOCCUS)

Organism: Gram-positive coccus

Specimen Collection: Blood culture, throat culture

Identification: Culture, rapid agglutination methods

Clinical Correlation: Clinically associated with a number of problems including pharyngitis, cellulitis, scarlet fever, puerperal infections, septicemia, hemolytic anemia, toxic shock–like syndrome, and the nonsuppurative sequelae of acute rheumatic fever and poststreptococcal glomerulonephritis

Suggested Reading

Cone LA, Woodard DR, Schlievert PM, Tomory GS. Clinical and bacteriologic observations of a toxic shock-like syndrome due to *Streptococcus pyogenes*. N Engl J Med 1987;317:146–149.

Dotters DJ, Katz VL. Streptococcal toxic shock associated with septic abortion. Obstet Gynecol 1991;78:549–551.

Silver RM, Heddleston LN, McGregor JA, Gibbs RS. Life-threatening puerperal infection due to group A streptococci. Obstet Gynecol 1992;79:894–896.

Whitted RW, Yeomans ER, Hankins GD. Group A beta-hemolytic streptococcus as a cause of toxic shock syndrome. A case report. J Reprod Med 1990;35:558–560.

SURFACTANT ALBUMIN RATIO

Specimen Collection: Amniotic fluid

Reference Range: A value of 50 mg/g or greater is predictive of lung maturity.

Clinical Correlation: This automated assay has the benefit of rapid analysis (30 minutes). Studies have shown good correlation with lecithin/sphingomyelin ratio and phosphatidylglycerol determinations.

Suggested Reading

Herbert WN, Chapman JF, Schnoor MM. Role of the TDx FLM assay in fetal lung maturity. Am J Obstet Gynecol 1993;168:808–812.

Russell JC, Cooper CM, Ketchum CH, et al. Multicenter evaluation of TDx test for assessing fetal lung maturity. Clin Chem 1989;35:1005–1010.

Steinfeld JD, Samuels P, Bulley MA, Cohen AW, Goodman DBP, Senior MB. The utility of the TDx test in the assessment of fetal lung maturity. Obstet Gynecol 1992;79:460–464.

TESTOSTERONE

Specimen Collection: Serum

Reference Range: Total 0.1–0.75 ng/mL

Clinical Correlation: For clinical correlations see the following chapters:

1. Amenorrhea (Chapter 18)
2. Hyperandrogenism (Chapter 20)
3. Hypothalamic Dysfunction (Chapter 21)
4. Ambiguous Genitalia (Chapter 12)
5. Oral Contraceptives (in relation to sex hormone-binding globulin; Chapter 25)

THEOPHYLLINE

Specimen Collection: Serum or plasma

Peak and trough levels are measured. The timing of the blood specimen for peak level depends on the medication.

Therapeutic Range: 10–20 µg/mL (56–111 µmol/L)

Clinical Correlation: Toxicity may occur at lower levels in pregnancy (See Chapter 7 on reproductive toxicology).

Patients with a low serum albumin level have an increased active (unbound) theophylline concentration.

Toxicity may be manifested by nausea, vomiting, diarrhea, arrhythmias, and seizures.

THROAT CULTURE

Specimen Collection: Swab specimen, avoid tongue and uvula

Clinical Correlation: Throat cultures obtained by the Ob-Gyn clinician may be sought for:

1. Streptococcal infection (group A β-hemolytic)
2. *Neisseria gonorrhoeae*

Gram-stained smears for N gonorrhoeae are not recommended due to the presence of other *Neisseria* species in the oropharynx.

Rapid screening tests for group A streptococci are widely available.

THROMBIN TIME

Specimen Collection: Sodium citrate tube

Reference Range: Normal range is usually within 5 seconds of the control value.

Clinical Correlation: Thrombin time has been used by some in screening for evidence of disseminated intravascular coagulation. This test is a reflection of both the qualitative and quantitative aspects of fibrinogen. It is prolonged in the following situations:

1. Low levels of fibrinogen
2. Dysfibrinogenemias
3. Patients on heparin
4. Presence of fibrin degradation products
5. Uremia

THYROID TESTING

Specimen Collection: Serum

Tests and Reference Ranges

Thyroxine (T_4)	5.0–12.6 µg/dL	(64–162 nmol/L)
Free thyroxine (free T_4)		
Equilibrium dialysis	1.6–2.4 ng/dL	(21–31 pmol/L)
Triiodothyronine (T_3)	90.0–190.0 ng/dL	(1.4–2.9 nmol/L)
Free triiodothyronine (free T_3)		
Equilibrium dialysis	125–300 pg/dL	(1.9–4.6 pmol/L)
T_3 uptake	25–35%	
Free thyroxine index (FTI)	1–4.3	
Thyroid-stimulating hormone (TSH)	0.5–3.8 µU/mL	(0.5–3.8 µU/L)
Thyroglobulin antibodies	Negative	
Thyroid microsomal antibodies	Negative	
Thyrotropin receptor antibodies (TRAb)	Negative	

Clinical Correlation: In general, the most significant recent laboratory advancement in thyroid testing has come with the development of sensitive TSH analyses that allow for evaluation of both hypothyroid and hyperthyroid dysfunctions. Thus, initial testing with TSH provides a great deal of information to the clinician. TSH testing in some laboratories has about the equivalent expense of the thyroid profiles that include T_4, T_3, T_3 uptake and FTI. Some of these TSH assays can detect values as low as 0.02 μU/mL. Patients with hyperthyroidism show levels in the 0.05–0.10 μU/mL range.

Low TSH levels will also detect secondary hypothyroidism.

Many of the thyroid tests are affected when a patient is ill or taking certain medications such as corticosteroids and dopamine. The TSH can also be suppressed to some degree in these situations.

The FTI has been used historically in pregnant patients due to the thyroglobulin-binding hormone changes that affect T_4 and T_3 uptake testing. This index generally works well in most patients unless there are marked abnormalities in the binding proteins or the patient is ill. Sensitive TSH determinations are supplanting use of FTI.

Free T_3 is used in assessing the rare patient with T_3 toxicosis.

In early pregnancy free thyroid hormone levels are elevated and TSH is decreased. This is thought to be secondary to human chorionic gonadotropin (1,2).

Thyroid microsomal antibodies have been found in about 20% of healthy women. They have also been identified in many women who manifest postpartum thyroid dysfunction.

Thyrotropin receptor antibodies (3) have primarily been used during pregnancy to predict neonatal thyroid dysfunction in patients with Graves' disease.

Other clinical correlations for thyroid testing are found in the following chapters:

1. Amenorrhea (Chapter 18)
2. Hypothalamic Dysfunction (Chapter 21)
3. Oral Contraceptives (Chapter 25)

References

1. Kennedy RL, Darne J. The role of hCG in regulation of the thyroid gland in normal and abnormal pregnancy. Obstet Gynecol 1991;78:298–307.
2. Kimura M, Amino N, Tamaki H, Mitsuda N, Miyai K, Tanizawa O. Physiologic thyroid activation in normal early pregnancy is induced by circulating hCG. Obstet Gynecol 1990;75:775–778.
3. Matsuura N, Konishi J, Fujieda K, et al. TSH-receptor antibodies in mothers with Graves' disease and outcome in their offspring. Lancet 1988;1:14–17.

TOXICOLOGY SCREEN

Specimen Collection: Blood (serum or EDTA), urine

Methodologies: Immunoassays, chromotography, spectrophotometry

Clinical Correlation: Testing commonly analyzes for amphetamines, anticonvulsants, analgesics, sedatives, narcotics, antidepressants, volatile substances, antihistamines, and drugs of abuse.

Ob-Gyn physicians may become involved with this testing during a pregnancy or have patients requiring testing secondary to overdose, etc. See also Chapter 7 on reproductive toxicology.

Suggested Reading

Hadi HA, Hill JA, Castillo RA. Alcohol and reproductive function: a review. Obstet Gynecol Surv 1987;42:69–74.

Melkonian R, Baker D. Risks of industrial mercury exposure in pregnancy. Obstet Gynecol Surv 1988;43:637–641.

Rosenak D, Diamant YZ, Yaffe H, Hornstein E. Cocaine: maternal use during pregnancy and its effect on the mother, the fetus, and the infant. Obstet Gynecol Surv 1990;45:348–359.

Wolman I, Niv D, Yovel I, Pausner D, Geller E, David MP. Opioid-addicted parturient, labor, and outcome: a reappraisal. Obstet Gynecol Surv 1989; 44:592–597.

Toxoplasma gondii

Organism: Protozoan

Specimen Collection: Maternal serum, fetal serum (cordocentesis)

Organism Identification

Serology—Sabin-Feldman dye test, indirect fluorescent antibody testing
Culture of fetal blood may reveal the organism
Molecular diagnostics—Polymerase chain reaction (PCR) assay has been developed (1).

Clinical Correlation: See Chapter 6 on fungal and parasitic infections.

Reference

1. Cazenave J, Forestier R, Bessiers M, Broussins B, Begueret J. Contribution of a new PCR assay to the prenatal diagnosis of congenital toxoplasmosis. Prenat Diag 1992;12:119.

TRANSFERRIN

Specimen Collection: Serum, fasting specimen

Reference Range: 200–400 mg/dL (2.0–4.0 g/L)

Clinical Correlation: Transferrin is an iron transport protein. It is elevated in iron deficiency anemia.

For use in nutritional evaluation see Chapter 27 on laboratory alterations in the management of gynecologic malignancies.

Treponema pallidum

Organism: Bacterial spirochete

Methodologies

Darkfield Examination

Specimen Collection: Notify microbiology laboratory in advance, clean earliest appearing lesion with saline, abrade surface, express serum and apply to slide, coverslip, examine with darkfield microscopy.

Organisms may occasionally be found in the skin lesions and lymph nodes in secondary syphilis.

Identification: Organisms are slightly larger than the diameter of a red cell, show rapid motion (flexing and rotation), and have a tight corkscrew appearance.

Clinical Correlation: Darkfield examination of oral and rectal lesions is less reliable due to the presence of nonpathogenic spirochetes.

RPR (Rapid Plasma Reagin)

Specimen Collection: Serum

Identification: RPR methodology uses charcoal and the identification of agglutination on a white plastic-coated card. The test is commonly done with unheated serum as opposed to the VDRL, which uses heat-inactivated serum.

VDRL (Venereal Disease Research Laboratory)

Specimen Collection: Serum, cerebrospinal fluid (CSF)

Identification: This is a flocculation test used to detect reagin (antibody to nontreponemal cardiolipin antigen)

Clinical Correlation: Used in screening for syphilis

Quantitative testing (VDRL titers) are used in evaluation of therapeutic response. VDRL titers should revert to low levels within 6–12 months following the initiation of therapy. Titers are recommended monthly during pregnancy and every 3 months when the patient is not pregnant. Initial monthly follow-up titers are also performed in patients who are HIV positive.

Positive test requires confirmatory testing (ie, FTA-ABS, MHA-TP)

The VDRL will become positive in 90% of cases 2–6 weeks following the appearance of the chancre. Because of the initial delay, darkfield examination is important for evaluation of chancres.

VDRL positivity in CSF is diagnostic of neurosyphilis, but the test can be negative in some cases of tabes dorsalis. Additional CSF findings include pleocytosis and elevated protein.

Serologic testing for syphilis is performed at the first prenatal visit and in some high-risk patients additionally in the third trimester.

False positive tests may occur in:

malaria	systemic lupus erythematosus
hepatitis	infectious mononucleosis
pregnancy	rheumatoid arthritis
narcotics abuse	

MHA-TP (Microhemagglutination—Treponema pallidum)

Specimen Collection: Serum

Reference Range: Usually < 1:160

Clinical Correlation: This is a confirmatory test for syphilis. It is not used for therapeutic monitoring because it remains positive.

False positives may occur in autoimmune disease and mononucleosis. It may be less sensitive than FTA-ABS in primary disease.

FTA-ABS (Fluorescent Treponemal Antibody-Absorption)

Specimen Collection: Serum

Identification: An indirect immunofluorescent test using killed *Treponema*

Clinical Correlation: This is a confirmatory test for syphilis, used following a positive VDRL or RPR.

False positives can occur with autoimmune disease, pregnancy, and drug addiction.

This test cannot be used for therapeutic monitoring because it remains reactive indefinitely.

Suggested Reading

Davis LE, Schmitt JW. Clinical significance of cerebrospinal fluid tests for neurosyphilis. Ann Neurol 1989;25:50–55.

Hart G. Syphilis tests in diagnostic and therapeutic decision making. Ann Intern Med 1986;104:368–376.

Trichinella spiralis

Organism: Nematode

Specimen Collection: Peripheral blood, creatine phosphokinase, lactic dehydrogenase, transaminases, serum, muscle biopsy

Identification: Eosinophilia, elevated enzymes, numerous serologic tests (bentonite flocculation) are test commonly used

Clinical Correlation: See Chapter 6 on fungal and parasitic infections.

Trichomonas vaginalis

Organism: Anaerobic flagellated protozoan

Specimen Collection and Identification: Place vaginal specimen on slide, mix with saline, and examine for motile trichomonads. Organisms may be more quiescent on cold slide.

Clinical Correlation: See Chapter 13 on vulvovaginitis.

TRIGLYCERIDES

Specimen Collection: Serum, 12–14 hours fasting, avoidance of alcohol for 3 days

Reference Range: 50–150 mg/dL (0.6–1.7 mmol/L)

Clinical Correlation: Triglycerides are used in the evaluation of hyperlipidemias and pancreatitis. Triglyceride is also used in the calculation of low-density lipoprotein cholesterol. Triglyceride levels are increased in pregnant patients and women taking oral contraceptives (see Chapter 25 on oral contraceptives).

TYPE AND CROSSMATCH

Specimen Collection: Serum

Procedures: Typing (ABO)
Rh (+/−)
Major crossmatch tests compatibility between donor's red blood cells and recipient's serum.
Minor crossmatch tests compatibility between donor's serum and recipient's red blood cells.
Agglutination indicates incompatibility.

Clinical Correlation: Recent administration of dextran and intravenous contrast media can affect the results. These can produce aggregation that appears similar to agglutination.

TYPE AND SCREEN

Procedure: Type, Rh, antibody screen

Clinical Correlation: Type and screen procedures are adequate for most operative procedures in Ob-Gyn. Type and cross is performed for obstetric cases in which severe bleeding is more likely and for radical surgical cases in gynecologic oncology.

UMBILICAL CORD BLOOD GASES

Specimen Collection: Aspiration of arterial/venous blood from umbilical cord, place on ice for immediate transportation to laboratory

Reference Range*
Umbilical arterial values (range)

pH	7.15–7.43
pCO_2	31.1–74.3 mm Hg
pO_2	3.8–33.8 mm Hg
Bicarb	13.3–27.5 mEq/L

Umbilical venous values (range)

pH	7.24–7.49
pCO$_2$	23.2–49.2 mm Hg
pO$_2$	15.4–48.2 mm Hg
Bicarb	15.9–24.7 mEq/L

Clinical Correlation: Clinically used to assess for metabolic, respiratory, and mixed acidemia. Some institutions routinely use this testing after all deliveries.

Reference

1. Yeomans ER, Hauth JC, Gilstrap LC 3d, Strickland DM. Umbilical cord pH, PCO$_2$, and bicarbonate following uncomplicated term vaginal deliveries. Am J Obstet Gynecol 1985;151:798–800.

* Values derived from Yeomans and colleagues (1).

URIC ACID

Specimen Collection: Serum

Reference Range: 2.2–5.7 mg/dL (0.13–0.34 mmol/L)

Clinical Correlation: Uric acid is decreased in normal pregnancy during the first and second trimester. The level then rises in the third trimester back to nonpregnancy levels.

Uric acid is elevated in many conditions where there is cell injury. It is the end product of purine metabolism. The main use of uric acid in Ob-Gyn has been in preeclampsia. The correlation of hyperuricemia with preeclampsia is described in Chapter 2 on hypertension.

URINALYSIS

Specimen Collection: Clean voided specimen to avoid vaginal fluid contamination

Refrigeration is recommended if there is transport delay. Refrigeration may occasionally precipitate crystals.

Reference Range

Specific gravity	1.015–1.030
pH	5.0–7.0
Protein	Negative
Ketones	Negative
Glucose	Negative
Red blood cells	0–5/high power field
White blood cells	0–5/high power field
Nitrite	Negative
Leukocyte esterase	Negative
Epithelial cells	Few
Casts	None to rare hyaline
Crystals	Negative

Clinical Correlation: See Chapter 16 on urine evaluation.

URINE CULTURE

Specimen Collection: Clean voided or catheterized specimen, send to the laboratory as soon as possible, avoid having specimen sit at room temperature

Reference Range: Most bacterial counts below 10,000/mL from clean voided specimens are considered contaminants.

Clinical Correlation: See Chapter 16 on urine evaluation.

VANCOMYCIN

Specimen Collection: Serum, peak is 30 minutes following dose, draw trough immediately prior to dosing.

Toxic Range: Toxicity may occur at levels > 30 µg/mL (20 µmol/L).

Clinical Correlation: Nephrotoxicity appears less now than with prior preparations. Ototoxicity can also occur.

This medication is used for methicillin-resistant staphylococci and for *Clostridium difficile.*

Suggested Reading

Ingerman MJ, Santoro J. Vancomycin. A new old agent. Infect Dis Clin North Am 1989;3:641–651.

VARICELLA-ZOSTER VIRUS (VZV)

Organism: Double-stranded DNA virus

Transmission/Incubation: Transmitted by respiratory droplets; incubation 13–17 days

Specimen Collection
Culture—vesicle fluid or material swabbed from the base of fresh lesions
Direct immunofluorescence—cell preparation on glass slide, air dry
Serology—red top tube

Results
Culture—Turnaround time varies with preparation (1–14 days). Shell vial method may yield results in 2–5 days.

Direct immunofluorescence with monoclonal antibody is the current method of choice over other direct methods and culture. Results usually take less than one hour to perform.

Fourfold titer increase is needed to diagnose infection. Enzyme-linked immunosorbent assay and fluorescent antibody to membrane antigen are used.

Clinical Correlation: Approximately 95% of women of childbearing age in the United States have serologic evidence of past VZV infection.

Serology is primarily used to assess if a patient is not immune (to guide maternal therapy with immunoglobulin [VZIg] if exposure has occurred).

VITAMIN B$_{12}$

Specimen Collection: Serum, fasting preferred

Reference Range: 200–900 pg/mL (148–666 pmol/L); result < 100 pg/mL is considered deficient, 100–200 pg/mL is borderline.

Clinical Correlation: Test results are used in conjunction with folate levels to evaluate macrocytic anemia.

WET MOUNT EXAMINATION (WET SMEAR)

Specimen Collection and Clinical Correlation: See the following chapters:

1. Vulvovaginitis (Chapter 13)
2. Bacterial Infections (Chapter 5)
3. Sexual Assault (Chapter 15)

Index